winter body

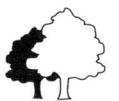

summer soul

The text of this book is composed in Rockwell, a 1933 design from Monotype, supervised by Frank Hinman Pierpont.

Printed by Creative Printing and Design
Hollister, Missouri

Cover by Flavie Mirat Lear, Flavie Productions

First Edition 2008
Second Impression 2009
ISBN 978-0-9771151-2-9

"Even in the midst of winter, I knew there lay
within me an invincible summer."
- Albert Camus

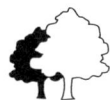

For Bill, Matthew, and Daniel. It is their love that kept me going,
even in the midst of winter. It is also my gift to the women of
courage who battle through this cancerous blizzard to find the
soft touch of a summer breeze dancing in their souls.

Chapter One

In the beginning:
nausea, baldness, lack of lashes;
pain in your soul so strong;
vulnerability, loss of confidence;
betrayal of the body, despair of the soul;
DEATH – watching, reaching.
So begins the nightmare.
I'm helpless as it unfolds.

Ovarian cancer.

With that diagnosis the nightmare begins.

I wake up from surgery with Bill leaning over me. He kisses me and says, "It's cancer." The gentle tones of his voice bleed with the sadness I see in his eyes.

Our son Daniel is there.

My brother Laird, his wife, daughter, and my sister Gail are there.

And Mom.

The tedium and toil of the five-hour surgery lie on their faces. While I sleep in a drug-induced womb with a man in white slicing out all my womanness, they wait with fear. With one look, I know the worst.

The fear of dying attacks me. They hover by my bed but I am looking at them through a glass wall. The unspoken word separates us.

I am alone and afraid.

Dr. Benson, my OBGYN, comes into the room. He tells me I will have a new doctor, Al Bonebrake, a gynecological oncologist. Dr. Benson called him in to do the surgery when he realized it was cancer.

Dr. Bonebrake tells my family, "She will have to undergo chemotherapy."

My sister Gail asks, "Will she lose all her hair?"

"Yes, she will."

Gail heads for the store and brings back a goody bag. She pulls out a bright pink hat. She gives it to me with all the love of a sister trying to make things better. She doesn't know how seeing that hat adds to my fear and dismay. I see only my bald head.

In two days, I take my first walk outside the room and see Dr. Bonebrake's name on my door. I hate that. I consider ripping it off. His crazy name brands me as a cancer patient. He should be an orthopedist. I wish for broken bones instead of a raw and bloody gut.

I leave the hospital after five days and go home with a wealth of flowers and plants. It is a procession as I leave the hospital. I'm in a wheelchair with yellow daisies and pink roses perched gingerly on my lap. Bill pushes me, and an aide pushes two carts of flowers. With ferns at my feet, I'm strangling in a garden of goodness.

People applaud the flowers and offer to help as we weave our way to the front door. "Somebody sure has lots of friends," pipes a stocky, white-haired man. Yes, but Jesus isn't one of them.

Home and recuperating from the surgery, I look around my living and family rooms at the abundance of yellow, pink, and vivid blue petals that stand out in 3-D relief against my white walls. Gratitude and sadness wrestle in my heart over this generosity sent by friends.

I have an overwhelming urge to pick up all the plants, vase by vase, and smash them against the wall. I don't want to have them in my home. They remind me of this awful illness. I only want to weep and pray that this nightmare will end.

It didn't end there and it still goes on, seven years and eight months later. I will not try to deceive anyone and say that it has not brought incredible sadness to my life, but it has also been a gift.

Living with cancer is, for me, a story of both sorrow and joy.

Chapter Two

Our first grandchild is born two weeks after my radical hysterectomy on July 1, 2000. I weep when our son calls to tell us of Eliza's birth. I should be in Florida with them to hold and love this Eliza of the great black mop of hair. Instead, I am lying in my bed struggling to get strong enough to begin chemotherapy. However, the birth of this tiny new person in my life is so important. She is my lifeline of hope. I want to be alive to watch her grow up, to be there for her. These hopes will carry me through my worst days during the chemo.

I decide to write letters to Eliza in case I don't make it. I will tell her about my childhood, my grandparents, meeting her granddad and her dad when he was a boy. After all, they are the stories I will tell her if I survive— my legacy and gift if I do not.

I write my first story that is full of the pure joy of childhood. I call it, "Never Never Land."

> Dear Eliza,
> When I was growing up, my grandmother Boyd and my granddad Pa lived in a white frame house at 212 Reagan Street in Pineville, Louisiana. It had a long screened in front porch with a green swing, and a green wicker sofa and chair.

Green plant stands topped with trailing spidery ferns stood by the front door waiting to grab me as I ran by. Japonica bushes, gardenias, and multi-colored irises partied all over their yard.

The fragrance of those blossoms embraced that porch. I can smell it on the breeze when I think of them. Everyone who walked by spoke to them as they sat on the swing or rocking chair. I thought they knew everyone, white or black, in that small southern town. My mother said they did.

Boyd would wave her flowered fan across her face. She asked us, "How do you children stand this heat?" I don't think it bothered me. I do remember the thick feel of the air against my skin. I felt part of the earth. If you went to the back of their house, you would find a set of stairs. Those stairs led to an attic that took you straight to Never, Never Land.

Gail, Dunn, and I would head for that attic as fast as our feet could take us. It was a long shadowy room that had a small window at the front. A bed and dresser stood as sentinels silently waiting for our return.

My grandparents used to let soldiers stay there if they needed a place during World War II. Old uniforms and dresses hung on a clothesline rope of make-believe galore. They gave off a musty smell that was perfume to us.

That attic was full of treasures—an old sword in its scabbard for my brother, and necklace loops of amber beads and Rita Hayworth earrings in shiny blues and greens for my sister and me.

A tiny Japanese blue and white tea set sat elegantly on a table. Its homely neighbor was a miniature green cast-iron stove complete with pots and pans.

A Shirley Temple doll surveyed her parlor with ageless and silent grace. I could be Wendy or Tinker Bell or transform into Betty Grable with a swish of a scarf or the click of an oversized earring on a small pink ear.

But best of all, we had this magic attic all to ourselves. Our mom never came up those stairs. If she had, that sword would have been long gone. My brother might have been, too.

Mom's voice drew us back when it was time for dinner.

Eliza, I've kept a battered Luke Skywalker, worn Batman comic books, a Ginny doll, and a small green cast-iron stove. If you go to the bottom of my basement stairs—well, Eliza, I'll make you a promise. I won't call you until dinner.

Love,

Grandma.

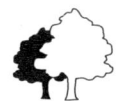

Chapter Three

It is five weeks after my surgery. We board a plane in Fayetteville, Arkansas, and fly to Pensacola, Florida. I step off the plane. Kerri is holding Eliza. She hands her to me. I can't keep from weeping. Johnson's Baby Shampoo fills my nostrils.

Eliza smells like hope.

I parade around the baggage carousel and proclaim to total strangers, "This is my granddaughter. This is the first time I've seen her."

I feel joy touched with fear. Will I live to see that mop of hair turn into a ponytail?

I hold my granddaughter every moment I am able. Her warm, fresh body gives me strength. I talk to my son about this baby, not about the upcoming chemotherapy. I want to forget it.

The week of reprieve is over. We get back on the plane and head to Missouri. For the first time, I don't want to see my home. It means one thing: begin chemotherapy.

I check into St. John's Hospital in Springfield, Missouri the next morning. My chemo regimen is a 24-hour drip administered in the hospital. I will have eighteen treatments. They will take place every three weeks.

At 6:30 a.m. a tall lean surgeon cuts into my left chest and installs a port. The chemo will invade my body there instead of through the veins in my arm.

The surgeon looks at me. "I'm so sorry you have to do this. If they had only caught it sooner . . ." His tone makes me feel dead already.

I start chemo the same day.

It's an eerie feeling - almost like I am watching myself from the other side of the room. I see myself being hooked up to the IV. I feel the healing poison begin its journey in my veins. It stings. I try to visualize the liquid traveling throughout my body. I say to myself, "This will work. It has to work. Please, God, make it work. Someone wake me up from this nightmare." I look at Bill. He is trapped in the dream with me.

The nurses check on me all the time. They are kind, but I want out. My eyes can't leave the clock. I know exactly how long this will take.

I have another doctor now. My insurance does not pay as well for Dr. Bonebrake. I refuse to give him up completely. He agrees to work with an oncologist at St. John's. Dr. Goodwin, my new doctor, stops by to read my chart. He is a short, gray-haired man in his middle sixties. He is wearing a v-neck vest and glasses. He looks more like an English professor than an oncologist. What he lacks in bedside manner he makes up for in brains. My cancer won't shrink from his compassion, but it will shudder from the medicines he prescribes.

Day becomes night. Bill stays with me the whole time. He sleeps on an uncomfortable recliner by my bed. I cannot make it without him. He is my rock.

Finally, I can go home. We get into my green Lexus. Everything is the same—the car, the drive, the house—all except me. I am different.

I am sick. I mourn the lost me, the healthy one who knows nothing of cancer. I know she will never be back. But I don't know that I will slowly become wiser and stronger.

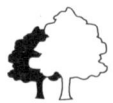

Chapter Four

This first regimen of chemo lasts from August until December. I check into the hospital every three weeks to receive the chemo. My entire body hates these days.

The bubbly blond nurse pops into my room. "You look too good to be getting chemo. We've dubbed you our chemo poster girl."

"You've got to be kidding."

I move to the hallway wrapped in my shapeless blue and white hospital gown. I grasp one side so my bottom doesn't grace the hallways. My other hand clings to the pole of my IV stand.

We are inseparable as we pace the hallways.

I return to my room. A different me looks back from my mirror—thin and sad. But I also see determination—to escape the hospital smell, the sadness and the chemotherapy poster girl.

I return home and feel okay at first but become more nauseated as the days pass.

A substitute counselor sits in my office at Reeds Spring High School. The quiet in my house is so loud I can't hear my own thoughts.

I can't breathe.

Bill is back at the courthouse. He is the Associate Circuit Judge in Stone County. He lives in a world of civil, juvenile, criminal and probate law. He is a problem solver, but he can't solve mine.

I prepare for losing my hair by buying two wigs. My friend Luann, who has beautiful thick hair, goes with me. My shoulder length hair isn't long for this world. I decide to get it cut before it falls out.

Luann immediately announces that she will get hers cut also so I won't have to do this alone. I weep. Her gentle goodness touches my heart. I don't quite understand it, but I'm beginning to receive one of the gifts of cancer.

Love and friendship will not leave me to face my nightmare in solitary confinement.

We have our hair cut on a bright, sunny day by two different stylists. Mine actually looks fine. Hers is a disaster. As we walk out of the shop, Luann says to me, "I look like I have a mushroom cloud on top of my head."

She does, and we burst into laughter and giggle all the way home.

How many women would laugh at such a miserable haircut? She's the only one I know. When I drop her off, her husband Gary is in the front yard. "Wow, Lu, atomic bomb!"

The next day she makes an appointment with a different stylist.

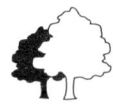

Chapter Five

These four months are the worst of my life. My hair begins to fall out—hair on my shoulders, hair on my pillow. Hair blankets any chair I sit in. I cry.

In Tulsa, my sister and I go shopping in the posh part of town. I try on a blue cotton pullover. It is covered in hair. I look at all the other women shopping and wish for their hair—hair that isn't coming out in wads.

After that trip, I have my head shaved and get my special order wig. I spend $300 on it. Bill waits in the outer room of the beauty shop because I can't bear for him to see me. The cosmetologist puts the wig on my head. It is all I can do not to cry in front of her. I look like an old lady—the ones you see in church with the prissy cuts and too short bangs. I can't imagine them in bed with anyone.

I will not be their clone.

Bill takes me for a sandwich. I am certain every person in McAllister's Deli knows I am wearing a wig. I swear to him, "I will never wear this wig again." I throw it in the closet and get out two cheaper ones I bought earlier.

I know that in the grand scheme of things losing my hair is minor, but it really bothers me. It assails my sense of being a woman. I've lost my dignity. I stand in front of the mirror in the bathroom after having my head shaved, then take off the wig, my husband right beside me.

I feel like a concentration camp survivor.

I put my face in my hands and weep. Bill takes me in his arms and says, "You are beautiful with or without your hair." I have never loved him more than at this minute. He gives me back my femininity. In this moment, I receive another gift of love that will not leave me throughout my ordeal.

In time, I write my own version of being hairless:

> ***"Ode to Baldness"***
> *Without my locks, I now look holy*
> *like a nun in a Barbie body.*
> *Okay, maybe I'm not so stacked as Barbie,*
> *but I've got the smooth, shiny limbs down pat.*
> *I save at the salon – no high dollar cut.*
> *No shampoo, no conditioner.*
> *The dollars are hanging in my pocket.*
> *Bald eyes – naked eyelids,*
> *invisible eyebrows.*
> *No mascara needed.*
> *Where would I put it?*
> *Hairy underarms - not for this Barbie babe.*
> *Couldn't find a hair with a microscope.*
> *Bring on the swimsuits and sundresses.*
> *It's year round summer under these pits.*
> *Bikini wax – no problemo.*
> *I am bare – no pubic hair.*
> *Sleek, skinny legs – throw out the razors*
> *and shaving cream. I too can have the hairless*
> *head and body of an Olympic swimmer.*
> *Wigs, wigs, wigs, I can have all I want,*

any color, any style – Goodbye Gray!
My hair is never out of place.
The bright-eyed young thing behind the counter said,
"What a great cut! Where do you get your hair done?"
"Honey chile, you don't want to know."

I lose about 20 pounds during those 18 weeks.

I don't actually vomit that often; the third and fourth days after chemo are the worst. I feel queasy all the time. I make myself walk in the park every day, determined to stay as strong as I can. I love to play tennis and want to be able to continue to play.

In a long line of sad, routine days, I never feel quite right.

One Saturday morning stands out clearly. Bill loves to hunt with our friend Paul. They decide to scout the woods to look for signs of deer. It is fall, and mist hangs in the air. Paul and his wife Maude pick us up. We drive down the hillside on a rough path with bushes scraping the sides of the truck. We stop in a clearing with cedar trees reaching up on every side. As we walk, it feels surreal. I seem to be there feeling slightly nauseous, but almost having an out of body experience. I am watching myself and feeling so much sadness for Bill and myself. I feel removed from the three of them as if they represent life and I death. The glass wall slides into place, separating us as we talk. They don't know I feel so encased in my aloneness.

When we leave, Maude gives me a jar of her homemade comfort soup. The glass wall cracks with her gesture. Her comfort in a jar warms my bones.

And then there is the part about my job, the job I embrace with my soul and my intellect. Education is my career life. I have taught every age from pre-school through college. I believe in the old Chinese proverb: "If you are planning for a year, sow rice; if you are planning for a decade, plant trees; if you are planning for a lifetime, educate your child." I am the junior/senior counselor at Reeds Spring High School. It is my passion to help young people discover their strengths and their immeasurable individual worth. I once had a parent conference with a mom whose son was perennially on the bad behavior list at school. The first words out of my mouth to her were, "I like your son. He has a great sense of humor." His mom looked at me in complete silence for several moments. "You are the first teacher I have ever met who said something positive about my son." I knew I had something valuable to give to my students.

Several years earlier, a counselor I worked with died from breast cancer. She worked until two weeks before she died. She looked like a living ghost to me, and her sadness permeated the building. I don't want to do that, so I take a leave of absence.

In January, I return to work, starting with half days. I dread wearing my wig to work, but everyone is great—students included.

In March, the big day comes when I throw out the wig. I pull it off as I drive home, so I decide to take the big plunge and leave the thing at home. My wigless maiden voyage is going to Red Lobster with Bill, Paul and Maude. They are supportive, telling me I look great.

School is next.

I dress carefully for my first day without my wig: big silver hoop earrings, a soft beige ribbed dress and wedge heels. Eyeliner and shadow are painstakingly applied. The first teacher I see says that I look like an ad for Vogue. It makes my day.

Chapter Six

A few months after finishing chemo, I notice a pain in my left thigh and swelling in my leg. I go straight to the doctor, and he sends me to the outpatient lymphedema clinic. I learn that when lymph nodes are removed during surgery, it upsets the flow of blood through the lymph system. The damage is permanent, as is the swelling.

I ask myself, "Is there no end to this?"

I meet Nora the nurse, a.k.a. the drill sergeant. She is tall and strong, and I do what she says.

Treatment involves having my leg wrapped completely in white bandages so often that I have to buy a pair of cheap tennis shoes two sizes larger than my regular shoes. I look like I have a mummy cast on my leg.

Sergeant Nora wraps my leg every day. The bandages stay on until the next day when she unwraps the leg. I go to the pool and have water therapy. Then, back to Nora for a leg massage and wrapping again. I follow this regimen for two weeks.

The two weeks end, and I now have to wrap my own leg at night and sleep in a long, padded sleeve. On top of that, I wear heavy, ugly support hose all the time, no matter the season. I loathe these hose. Nora tells me repeatedly that I must wrap the leg, sleep in the sleeve and wear the hose for the rest of my life. At first, I believe that, but as this illness tries to take more and more away from me, tiny seeds of determination are forming in my soul. They aren't fully sprouted yet, but they are planted.

My first rebellion with the hose comes with tennis. I wear the bloomin' things under my tennis skirt one Sunday afternoon. It is at least 85 degrees. Bill and I are playing mixed doubles. I have never been so hot in my life. A huge vein pops out on my left forehead. I call the answering service, and my doctor is on call. I say, "I think I might have a stroke." I tell him that I won't wear the hose for tennis. "Okay," he answers—more fertilizer for those seeds of determination I'm growing. I don't have to do everything the doctor tells me.

I am going to make my own decisions about my body.

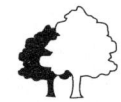

Chapter Seven

It's October 2001, and I'm in the gynecologist's office for my regular pelvic exam. It hurts. That bothers me. I call Dr. Bonebrake, and he orders blood work to see if it shows that the cancer is back. The blood work results are normal. A PET scan is next. One of the unpleasant realities of being a cancer patient is hurry-up-and-wait. I won't get the results until Monday.

Bill and I decide to go camping for the weekend on the Buffalo River in Arkansas. Trees are decked in gold with lingering green, and they envelop that wild, rushing river. We hike the mountain trails under cobalt blue skies with that iridescent river flowing below. I pray all the time that the test will be negative. In my heart, I know it will not. I am having some twinges in my pelvis every now and then that I can't explain. I lie in the tent at night with Bill sleeping beside me and imagine all the possibilities. I dread Monday.

Bill leaves for a judicial conference in St. Louis Monday morning. Dr. Bonebrake calls late that afternoon. The results are very bad—numerous spots of recurrence. Compassion and sadness flow from the receiver as he speaks.

He is disturbed that I am getting the news by myself.

I keep calling Bill, but the number at the hotel is busy. I call our sons, and they are very supportive, but I need Bill.

Finally, I call the hotel manager and ask if he could check Bill's room. Bill calls immediately. He is devastated by the report.

Bill arrives home the next day, and we meet with Dr. Bonebrake. He recommends chemo again. The prognosis is not good. When I hear these words, I feel horror move inside me. We leave his office and step into a beguiling sunny world—a world that I am being forced to leave by this demon cancer. My mortality is closing in on me.

I want to be anyone but me.

From the doctor's office, we drive straight to the high school where I work. We meet with the principal, my co-counselor, and the guidance secretary. I tell them that the cancer is back. I want to resign.

I know this battle is not a part-time job.

There is a certified counselor on staff who is available for my job. The principal doesn't want me to leave, but understands my situation. I have his support.

Bill and I go into my office and close the door. We pack 24 years of teaching and counseling in boxes and load them into our car. I pack away my thoughts as tightly as those boxes. If I don't, grief will overwhelm me.

We call our sons to tell them the news. As a mother, I want the best of worlds for our sons, and that world does not include a mom dealing with cancer. At the same time, I need to hear their words of support and love. Matt and Daniel help keep me in the fight.

Daniel is struggling with the decision of where to attend law school. For the past five years, he has been living in Nashville. He loves the city and has many close friends. He is trying to decide between the University of Missouri and the University of Tennessee.

Daniel comes home to Missouri to be closer to us during this difficult time. This decision is difficult for him financially because he is an in-state student in Tennessee and a tuition-paying student in Missouri. I will not forget this gift of love.

Chapter Eight

Bill and I opt for a second opinion. I collect all my records and scan films and hand carry them onto the plane to the MD Anderson Clinic in Houston, Texas. I manage to get an appointment with Dr. David Gershenson, one of the best ovarian cancer specialists in the country.

The MD Anderson complex is huge. We walk into the lobby of its hotel for patients and their families. Everywhere I look, women with hats or scarves on their heads look back at me with vulnerable, timid smiles.

Dr. Gershenson and a young resident examine me the first morning. We have a consult the next day. He agrees with everything Dr. Bonebrake said. Dr. Gershenson is very compassionate, yet has the saddest eyes.

He tells me that I will be on chemo for the rest of my life.

These words haunt me still, to this day. They also give me a sudden steely determination. This illness and I have now drawn the lines in the sand. The battle begins.

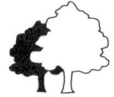

Chapter Nine

We fly home ready to face more treatments. Having resigned from my job, my priority now is my health. My only chance for survival is to wage a full assault against this deadly disease.

I receive two different types of chemo at Dr. Goodwin's office in Springfield. Chemo for three weeks, one week off, and chemo again. This schedule continues for three or four months.

The office waiting room is large, filled with patients with yellowed skin, bony arms and hopeless eyes. The nurse steps into the waiting room and shouts my name. It is somehow demeaning, like calling cattle being hauled in for slaughter. I step into the next room, and the nurse checks my vitals. She draws my blood so Dr. Goodwin can see if my counts are okay for treatment. If they aren't, I will have to turn around and go home until next week.

It's a drag because once I'm psyched up for the treatment, I want to get it over with and mark that time off my calendar. Plus, each time I'm sent home, it extends the time until I am through with the entire regimen. Believe me, the end date is something like high school graduation. I circle the date on my calendar, and it's what I live for every nauseous moment. I know when that date is reached, I will be through feeling bad, through with fifty-mile trips to Springfield, through with being stuck with needles in veins that are too small for this, through with losing my hair, and hopefully through with cancer. Graduation Day!

The blood work is good so I walk back to the chemo treatment room. This large, white room is crammed with sick-looking people seated in large plastic covered recliners. Each person is hooked to an IV on a pole that she can drag to the bathroom. There is absolutely nothing healing in the atmosphere in this room. It smells like sickness and chemicals.

I want to gag.

The nurses wave me to a chair. The blond one approaches me with her needles. I cringe. She tried to stick me last week and couldn't do it. She calls for Pat, who can hit anyone's veins. The TV is blaring, people are coughing, monitors screech and bleep. Next to me, a man with a yellow face makes conversation. The nurse stops by another recliner. I want to get started so I can get out. I look around the room and do not see hope or life. I just see sick people, myself included, all of us facing death.

I wonder which of us will go first.

Bill is in court, so my Aunt Ella takes me to most of these treatments. She sits beside me for however long it takes—usually four hours. She drives me to Springfield and back. I cannot thank her enough. Her love, care and concern help carry me through this sorrowful room to my vision of hope for a future.

Chapter Ten

Another PET scan shows three remaining spots of cancer. Bill and I decide to fly to Sloan Kettering Cancer Center in New York City. Once again, I collect records, films and scan reports.

My consult is with a young Asian-American doctor. He concurs with my Springfield doctors on the diagnosis but is more hopeful. He says that I can live for a long time with this, but I do need treatment. I tell him that I've started yoga lessons. He practices yoga himself.

We stay with my cousin Dave and his wife Susie. Dave takes us to dinner with one of Bill's cousins and an aunt. Bill's cousin Melissa mentions a friend whose father had brain cancer. His prognosis was to live six weeks. He consulted a nutritionist, changed his diet and was alive a year later. I ask her to e-mail me that nutritionist's name. I feel a sliver of hope creep into my mind.

Susie gives me a jar of arabinogalactin powder before we leave. Her doctor recommends it as a cancer preventive. He wrote the book on blood types, diet and cancer. I take the powder reluctantly, not convinced that it will help. I am touched by Susie's belief in its power. Getting to know Susie and spending time with Dave is another gift.

Chapter Eleven

We fly home. The e-mail arrives with the nutritionist's name—Dr. Jeanne Wallace. That name seems familiar. I get out the report I had ordered from the Health Resources Corporation, Jan Guthrie's company in Conway, Arkansas. She is a 20 plus-year survivor of stage IV ovarian cancer. She was featured in the Wall Street Journal several years ago in an article about people who survive difficult cancers.

I get to know Jan on the phone and then meet her for lunch. She is an inspiration. She is the living proof for me that it can be done. Cancer does not always win. Jan is not cancer free, but she has lived with it for more than 20 years. I can handle that.

My report from Jan's company contains the latest clinical research and treatment programs in the United States and abroad. It also has a section on alternative medicine. I thumb through those pages. The name jumps off the page—Dr. Jeanne Wallace, Ph.D. in clinical nutrition. I can't ignore the coincidence. I call Jan. "Do you know anything about this woman, this Dr. Wallace?" Jan doesn't hesitate. "She knows more about ovarian cancer and diet than anyone in the United States." That is enough for me.

I call Dr. Wallace's office. Her assistant Michelle asks that my doctor send them a copy of my pathology reports from my original surgery. Dr. Bonebrake's nurse sends the lab reports. Dr. Wallace reads those reports and then develops my regimen of supplements and recommends a diet.

Bill and I schedule our first phone consult with Dr. Wallace. She lives in North Logan, Utah, so we decide to forego an office visit. Bill is not 100% behind this nutritional idea. He has a mechanical engineering degree as well as his JD in law. His rational, scientific mind balks at this unapproved non-medical treatment. He goes along with it because it gives me hope.

When Dr. Wallace calls, Bill and I get on the phone. The judge calls his first witness—Dr. Wallace. He rains questions. She answers every one. She isn't threatened. She knows her stuff! We hang up. Bill says, "I'm impressed." I think, high praise from this country judge in the Show-Me State.

My life changes with this phone call. Fried foods, sugar, alcohol, non-organic food of any kind, white flour, white rice, and white bread no longer live in comfort in my house. Broccoli appears on my table every day, as do piles of other fresh vegetables. I have a list of which kinds of fruit have the most sugar. I only eat those fruits once or twice a week. I don't drink fruit juice. It's loaded with sugar. I drink green tea by the gallon. I buy chickens and turkey from an area antibiotic-free farm. Our local blueberry farm, Persimmon Hill, keeps me supplied with blueberries and shiitake mushrooms. I eat grass-fed beef, fresh fish and the venison that Bill brings home during hunting season. Bill and I have one healthy diet! He is diabetic so this diet is great for him too.

I swallow 44 pills a day without complaint. They are the supplements Dr. Wallace prescribes to help boost my immune system. I feel stronger within weeks.

Your perspective changes when you want to stay alive. People ask me how I can stay on this diet. I answer, "How can I not?"

Dr. Wallace's premise is not that she can cure cancer. If I eat the most appropriate foods and support it with supplements, I can help my body stay strong. I can boost my immune system. If I have a new treatment, I'll be able to handle it. With ovarian cancer, there are recurrences. If I follow the diet, the recurrences will be spaced further apart. Dr. Wallace works in tandem with my medical treatment, not against it.

Chapter Twelve

"Tadasana, down dog, and namaste"—foreign words and thoughts until I begin to study yoga. Now they are a part of my soul. Yoga is another part of my assault upon the cancer in my body. My yoga teacher is Ginny Ross. She is an RN and has been practicing yoga for about 20 years. Picture a petite woman with short, gray hair and bright gentle eyes, and you can see Ginny. She has a tender, positive and loving soul. I feel its blessing every time I work with Ginny.

When I begin yoga, I have the stiffest and tightest body that Ginny has ever seen. Not that she tells me then. Nothing but positive words ever comes from Ginny Ross. From the moment I meet her, I never feel anything but warmth and encouragement. She begins my study of yoga with restorative poses. She doesn't want to stress or overtire my chemo-laden body. She begins by building my physical strength, and more importantly, my inner spiritual strength.

Ginny teaches yoga according to the philosophy of B.K.S. Iyengar. His book *Light on Life* is one of my spiritual guides. This philosophy is teaching me to live fully in the moment. As I deal with cancer, this idea is an incalculable help. Joseph Campbell has a saying I have taken to heart: "the world is full of sorrows, but you can choose to live in joy."

The sorrow of my world is cancer, but I choose to live in joy every day. That is how I avoid drowning in fear and sadness.

Yoga is a discipline for the body and the soul. I practice almost every day. I slowly get stronger and stronger. As my body does, so does my soul. I am so much more in tune with my body and its well being. When I was first diagnosed, I felt like my body had betrayed me. I didn't think this would ever happen to me. Through yoga, I learn to listen to my body, to have awareness in parts of my body that I have previously ignored.

Ginny always does a restorative pose at the end of my lessons. She puts me in a peaceful position. I lie there for about 15 minutes. Ginny reads positive quotes full of healing currents. We end the session by repeating, "All is well in our world." I leave yoga class with that feeling.

Once, Ginny talked to me about the cancer being a part of my body, and that I shouldn't treat dealing with it as a battle. I came up from my pose and said, "No way."

This is a battle for me, a battle for life, and I want to do anything I can to fight it with every breath. I want none of it left in my body.

Somehow, by practicing the physical part of yoga, I begin to feel stronger within myself. I know myself better and realize just how deep within myself I can go to tap that strength. I am beginning to have confidence in my body's and my soul's abilities to help me heal. I am strengthening my faith in myself and in God. As yoga puts me more in touch with myself, it links me ever closer to the universal oneness that all humans share. Without this illness, I don't think I would have ever studied yoga. Ginny, yoga and all its blessings are another gift.

I plan to follow this pathway for the rest of my life.

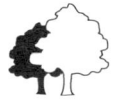

Chapter Thirteen

I still need to decide on a treatment. I call the National Cancer Institute and talk with one of their doctors. He suggests tamoxifen, as did Dr. Dizon at Sloan-Kettering. Dr. Goodwin and I decide to try this pill for two or three months. I have a CAT scan of my pelvis. The cancerous spots are not shrinking. Tamoxifen doesn't work for me. It's back to the drawing board.

Bill and I consult with Dr. Bonebrake. This tall, athletic man welcomes us with compassionate eyes. His intellect matches the prowess of his body. He wants me to beat this scourge.

We opt to step out of the box. Instead of chemotherapy again, we decide to try radiation on the remaining spots. First, Dr. Bonebrake wants to do a debulking surgery to remove every trace of cancer that he can find. He spends more than three hours scraping my guts.

I am barely back in my room after surgery before it is filled with family and friends. I am humbled by their love and hope for me.

Home in five days, I'm hurting but glad to be there. Bill gets me up and walking as soon as possible to speed my recovery. Dr. Bonebrake refers me to Dr. Drew Rogers in St. John's radiation oncology department. After scans and x-rays to be sure the cancer isn't spreading to my colon, Dr. Rogers is ready to give radiation a try.

Bill and I walk into the radiation clinic in Springfield. The receptionist says hello with a big smile. We sit down and fill in the necessary paperwork.

The reception room is small. Coffee, magazines and a TV are available. The intercom interrupts us with a polite, "Mrs. Kirsch, will you please report to the treatment room." What a difference from the chemo room. Here, I keep my dignity.

I walk back to the treatment area where a technologist intercepts me and escorts me to the radiation room. Becky treats me as a real human being, not a sickly patient. She instructs me on where to lie down and how to breathe. I pull my jeans halfway down my thighs, cover myself with a sheet and lie down on the table. Becky and the other techs spend several minutes making sure that my body is in the right position on the table. They leave the room.

I lie on the large, white machine that will deliver the radiation to the tumors. A voice tells me not to move. The machine moves around me shooting beams of radiation into my body. The heavy door opens, and the techs return to help me off the table. They don't know that their compassion and warmth are a part of my healing.

I complete six weeks of radiation. One spot of cancer remains. Dr. Rogers recommends an iridium implant. He is the only physician in Springfield who will try this procedure. It is risky because the potential for damage to my healthy organs is great.

I am not afraid. I trust this doctor and want to be healthy.

Dr. Rogers suffers from back pain. He is scheduled to have surgery the week after he performs my implant. Mine is the last surgery he ever does. He plans to retire after his own surgery due to his back problems. I'm lucky to have the chance to benefit from his experience.

To prepare for the implant, I must have measurements taken inside my pelvis. Fully alert, I lie on a table in the radiation clinic with two men and one woman putting tubes inside my body.

With total strangers' hands inside my pelvis, I learn humbleness from this illness.

During the procedure, I need to pass gas and cannot contain it. I am embarrassed and say, "I'm so sorry." The physicist immediately replies, "It is not your fault. You are not in control of yourself here." His response lets me "save face" and continue the ordeal. This illness and its treatment invade the very core of my body and my dignity. I can't feel uppity or snobbish doing something like that—Mrs. Judge or not!

Before I had this illness, I think I had the idea that since I was a basically good person, I didn't deserve to have something like cancer. I now know that nobody deserves this illness and that, as human beings, we are all worth the same. Cancer is a great leveler. It doesn't care if you are a president or a peasant; it will still come after you.

What matters is what you bring to the battle—heart, soul and steely determination.

Chapter Fourteen

Before I go to the hospital, I get a phone call from our son Matt. He tells me about Eliza. He talks about the way she cuddles her baby doll Sara. He tells me how she loves to sit on his lap while he reads to her. His voice quivers for an instant when he tells me that he sings her to sleep with "Swing Low, Sweet Chariot" and "You Are My Sunshine." Those are the songs I sang to him, and my daddy sang to me. My eyes get moist.

I cannot help but have special feelings for this sparkly-eyed two-year-old with her beyond-her-years wit and wisdom. I think she knows that I do. She seems to sense our unique connection.

Matt ends our conversation with this story. "Mom, Eliza and I were looking at a family album yesterday. When she got to your picture, she took it out of the album, kissed it, and slipped it back into place."

I can't speak for a moment. Tears of love spill down my cheeks. I feel the blessing of that kiss every day. I want years more of those kisses.

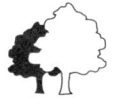

Chapter Fifteen

I check into the hospital. Dr. Rogers orders the iridium. Very strict regulations govern the use of this radioactive substance. The doctor cannot order the precise amount until the patient has been measured and is waiting for the medicine. I lie in the hospital waiting. Bill is with me. Time passes. I'm not sure if I have waited one or two days.

I am in surgery again. Dr. Rogers performs the implant. From surgery, I go to isolation. Bill is there on the other side of the door. He e-mails my friends and family to tell them how I am doing. He doesn't describe me as a cancer patient flat on my back. In Bill's lingo, I am one RED-HOT MAMA!! He can't wait to get me home.

The ceiling and I become close friends as I lie flat on my back for 52 hours. My bed is blocked off from the rest of the room. The smiling young faces of my tow-haired son and his curly-haired older brother crowd into my thoughts. I am glad I got to see them grow up.

I am not afraid. I concentrate on my will to live. I pray and think about our upcoming camping trip to Texas. The ethereal and the mundane dance together in my mind.

Only the nurse is supposed to come close. Bill comes in anyway and jokes that he might as well be radioactive too because we aren't planning any more babies!

Finally, another doctor and techs come to remove the tubes, and I am more than ready. There are over 188 iridium seeds in 23 ribbons encased in the tubes in my pelvis. They come out one by one. I am awake for this procedure. I am afraid it will hurt.

I lie absolutely still as they pull the tubes from my raw pelvis.

The medical team works with gentleness and encouragement. I bless them in my heart. Dr. Rogers is already in the hospital awaiting his surgery.

I am back in my room. I lose track of time but am ready to go home. Physically, I can barely stand to hoist myself into the front seat of our truck. Emotionally, I am floating high above the tan truck seat. I am so glad to be out of that hospital. We drive 10 minutes across town to my mother's and spend the night. I don't think I can sit on my bottom for the one-hour drive home.

Chapter Sixteen

Before I went into the hospital for the radiation treatment, we purchased a 24-foot travel trailer. Bill decided not to run for a fifth term as judge. He chose to spend his time with me. Five attorneys wanted his job. Every one of them came to his office and asked if he was running for reelection. They said that they wouldn't oppose him if he still wanted the job. They didn't want to add to our burdens. Possibly, they didn't think they could beat him. I saw that all lawyers aren't sharks. Some of them are country gentlemen.

The prospect of that first camping trip kept me going when I was flat on my back. We decide to head to South Padre Island, Texas. In one week, I go from the hospital bed to the trailer bed. I take my pillow, my joy of being free, and we roll down the open road.

Bill and I had always joked about RV's and the "old people" who drive them. Now, here we are joining that elite silver-haired group. I can hear my mother saying, "Never say you or your kids will never do anything. That is a guarantee that it will happen."

We park our RV in a park near the beach. We ride bikes and walk the beach. Our Springer spaniel, Jesse, is our companion for the trip. It is Jesse's first trip to the ocean. I should record it for posterity. We arrive at the beach as a slew of sea gulls welcomes us overhead. Jesse's birding instincts go into overdrive, and he hits the water like a rocket. He literally leaps across the waves bellowing at the top of his doggie lungs. He keeps bobbing and leaping for almost an hour. I guess hope springs eternal not only in the human breast. A crowd of beachgoers gathers to watch him and laughs at his antics.

Jesse personifies the joy of life in action.

That is how I feel on this trip. I am so excited to be alive that everything I do seems like a leap and, like Jesse's, my hope is eternally there—hope that I will never have to deal with this cancer again.

We leave South Padre and head for San Antonio. By this time, I'm desperately in need of a haircut. Any woman knows that it is just plain crazy to go to an unknown hairdresser in an unknown city, but this is what I do. While shopping, I admire a shop owner's haircut. I tell her about my cancer experience and that I need a new look. She picks up the phone and makes an appointment for me with George.

As I walk towards the salon, Bill says, "Don't let them color your hair." That is precisely what I have in mind, but I don't reply. He stays in the car with a book.

As soon as I enter, a diminutive gray-haired black lady swoops me in to wash my hair. She asks, "What we gonna do to this hair today?" I answer, "I am thinking about a new style and color." "Oh, no," she says. "You don't want to color this hair. This is too good-lookin'." She sends me to George.

George motions me into a sleek, black chair and asks the same question, "What are we going to do today?" I again say, "I'm thinking about a new style and color."

George looks at me, fluffs my hair, and says, "I could make a lot of money off you but I just can't color this hair. Women pay me to get hair this silver."

The woman in the next chair and her hairdresser say simultaneously, "Don't color that hair." I sit up straighter and eyeball myself in the mirror.

Okay, these compliments are nice but since everyone else is sporting a dye job, is it my job to make the rest of the world look younger?

When he finishes, George insists on walking me to the car to meet my husband. Bill's first comment: "I'm glad you didn't color your hair." I guess if Emmy Lou can keep hers silver, so can I. After all, it's hair—not a bald head.

Chapter Seventeen

It's February, and we are landing at Denver International Airport. Matt and Eliza meet us at the baggage claim. Eliza is unusually shy and doesn't run to us. She stays with me while the guys get the luggage, holding my hand. She looks up at me and says, "I love you, Grandma." I pick her up. "I love you, too, Eliza, so, so much." Her brown eyes sparkle and so does my heart.

We are here for the birth of our first grandson. I am excited and ready to see this baby boy come into the world. Kerri's mom was with her for Eliza's birth. I assume that I'll get the honor with Kai. My son tells us that Kerri wants him to be there—no one else.

I am devastated.

I still feel weak from the implant. Weepiness lies under the surface of all my thoughts. This new little boy means life to me. To see him enter this earth means that I will go on in that tiny, fresh human being. I need to see that moment of joy when life triumphs.

I am denied my moment. I feel betrayed. I am the second-class grandmother.

I don't think my son or his wife has any idea how important that moment is to me. I don't tell them. I realize that even the ones you love the most don't understand the despair of this illness. They can't. It isn't happening to them.

Kerri and I break down about this decision. She says it was her decision, not Matt's. As I weep, I admire her honesty. She doesn't come between my son and me. I no longer feel betrayed. I get to come into the hospital room 15 minutes after Kai is born. Kai is shiny, new, and he is my grandson. I hold him in my arms and cry. He and I both feel fragile on this earth.

I know my daughter-in-law had every right to choose who would see her son be born. I didn't get those choices when my sons were born. Bill was in Vietnam when Matt was born. The doc I had with Daniel didn't allow fathers in the delivery room. Perhaps, I wanted just once to have the people I loved with me at one of life's most special moments.

The raw truth: I wanted to shove my healthy grandson's tiny fist in death's face.

Kerri gives me the gift of my grandchildren all the time. We are the first ones to keep them overnight. I go to school with Eliza on the first day of school. She puts them on the phone to talk with us whenever we call. She encourages them to love and respect their grandparents. That is her gift. It is wrapped in the fresh, sweet voices of Eliza and Kai when they say I love you, Grandma. That is all I need.

Chapter Eighteen

At home, we pick up our lives in Kimberling City. I begin volunteering at our local library and Christian Associates. I play tennis every Wednesday night through all of this.

Six months later, I am in the bathroom looking at a toilet full of blood. I panic. I am in Dr. Bonebrake's office the next day. He does a pelvic exam. There is nothing abnormal inside me. The bleeding is a side effect of the radiation. It may continue for the rest of my life or happen periodically. I don't care as long as it isn't cancer.

Chapter Nineteen

It's a crisp October day, and we are driving to Columbia to see Daniel, who is trapped in the mind games of law school. We stop for gas. I get out of the car and feel a sharp pain in my right leg. I can hardly walk to the restroom. I get back into the car and dismiss the pain as a leg cramp.

After several days at Daniel's, we drive to Kansas City and board a plane for Sacramento. Fortunately, I wear support hose when I fly. We spend two days with a lifelong friend and head for San Francisco for a wedding. As I dress for the rehearsal dinner, I notice how swollen my leg is. I can barely put my shoe on my foot.

We arrive at the Beaulieu Vineyards in the Napa Valley. Wine flows, and old friendships are renewed. I ignore my leg.

Home again and another visit to the doctor. Techs perform an ultrasound on my leg. There is a clot. Both Dr. Goodwin and Dr. Bonebrake think it might be a normal occurrence of traveling until I have a second one in December. Now, I take coumadin. Every three days, I drive to Skaggs Hospital in Branson to get my blood tested to make sure the coumadin dose is correct.

This is a 15-mile drive each way. Taking my blood should be a minor ordeal, but my veins are so ruined by chemo that they don't like to cooperate. That means more than one stick per visit until I figure out which tech can do it right the first time.

Finally, Dr. Goodwin thinks we have the coumadin under control.

Chapter Twenty

Bill and I are ready to take off again and head for South Carolina with our travel trailer.

We spend the second night in the mountains of north Georgia in Red Rock State Park. I love the mountain scenery with the scent of pines invading our nostrils. We move to Augusta and weather the last of an ice storm. Pine boughs break and fall all night long.

Savannah is our next stop. We immerse ourselves in the thick Southern magic of this ethereal city. A bus tour produces a wealth of information about the city's Revolutionary War past.

My leg begins to swell again. I get my blood tested in each city and fax the results to Dr. Goodwin. I call his nurse for any changes in my coumadin dose.

Our next stop is Hunting Beach State Park in South Carolina. We park our RV with an unlimited view of the beach. We bike the trails and walk the shore. It's chilly, but we almost have the park to ourselves.

Hunting Beach is near Beaufort, of Forrest Gump fame. We tour the city with a retired physician who now owns a shrimp business. We play tennis, and my leg gets worse.

After a week, we move the RV to Charleston. We spend my birthday in the city and dine at the Cotton Club on shrimp and grits. I give myself a night off from my diet.

My leg is in the back of my mind. It is bothering me, but I don't want to ruin my birthday.

Cancer and its side effects constantly invade my life.

The next morning, we attend Sunday School in a nearby Methodist church. We like to meet some locals and get a feel for the area. We drive downtown after Sunday school to hear a sermon in the oldest Methodist church in Charleston. We stand to sing a hymn.

A sharp pain rips down my leg. I know I am in trouble.

We get back to the RV and dress for tennis. Who am I trying to kid? As we head for the courts, I tell Bill that we better make a detour for the hospital.

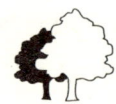

Chapter Twenty-One

A young doctor meets us in the emergency room at St. Francis Hospital. His kind voice tells me that I need to spend the night. I have blood clots in both legs. I expected one, but not both. Every time I meet a doctor, it is more bad news.

The aides wheel me to a regular room and tell me not to get up except to use the restroom. Dr. Carey Farber appears at my door. He introduces himself by saying, "I don't usually take patients like this, but the emergency room doctor is a good friend. He called and asked me to take care of you. My first question was, 'Is she one of the tribe?'"

Dr. Farber takes on this Gentile woman anyway and first checks on my diet. I don't remember the nurses or doctors in Springfield ever saying anything about diet and coumadin. I'm eating lots of collard greens and drinking gallons of green tea. Both of these have lots of vitamin K, which aids in the formation of clots. I'm working against myself and don't know it. I don't want to give up these foods because they are part of the diet I'm using to fight the growth of the cancer.

Dr. Farber puts me on Lovenox injections. I can continue on my diet with that medication. I have two ultrasounds on my legs. Dr. Farber recommends a CAT scan and installation of a Greenfield filter when I return home. He fears that the cancer has returned and is causing the clots. I don't want to hear that, but I don't forget it either.

Dr. Farber keeps me in the hospital for a week. He, Bill, and I have long discussions about life, movies, religion, etc. Bill and the doc go to a movie one night while I am glued to the hospital bed. Dr. Farber is our friend. He is one of the gifts of cancer.

I leave the hospital with strict instructions to ride all the way home with my legs elevated on pillows in the back seat. We drive to Orangeburg, South Carolina, with my family history in my hand. My ancestor, Lewis Golson, was given land grants in South Carolina for his service to the colonies as a captain in the militia. I want to see where my family came from so long ago.

It is Sunday, and nothing is open. We have coffee at Arby's and grab a phone book. A Lewis Golson is listed in the phone book. I call the number and a Southern-to-the-grits voice answers. I tell the elderly lady who I am and about my family history. She drawls back, "Honey, I am sure you are related to us. We have been 'heah forevah'."

We follow her directions to Golson Road and a tiny white Methodist church. We walk in the cemetery. I pass grave after grave marked Golson with Confederate soldiers lying in them as well as some from World War I. The lump in my throat surprises me. Maybe it shouldn't; I am touching my mortality with theirs.

Chapter Twenty-Two

We drive home, and of course, I'm back at the doctor's office. Unbelievably, they decide to put me back on coumadin. I don't trust my doctor's judgment about this issue. Every single time I am on coumadin instead of Lovenox, I get a clot. Coumadin should work, but it doesn't. April arrives. So does a clot, and one again in May.

Chapter Twenty-Three

My friend Luann is retiring from teaching kindergarten in May. I am determined to go to that celebration. Luann's mother died in February, and I wasn't able to travel to the funeral because of a blood clot. Our son Daniel went instead. Luann and I raised our children together. She feels like family.

My doctor says that I should not go to her retirement party. I tell Bill that I am going. I am not going to let those blood clots prevent me from being there for my friend who is always there for me.

We arrive at the high school for the party. My former principal brings out a rolling desk chair for me. Bill pushes me across the floor to a seat. I put my left leg up on another chair. I don't like feeling helpless in front of my colleagues and friends.

I'm glad to be there to share Luann's joy. Her friendship is a constant throughout my battle. She is a blessing in my life.

Chapter Twenty-Four

My 82-year-old mom has been struggling with her health the past two years. She has not been diagnosed with any serious problem, but I know she is failing. I sit in the living room with my mom. She tells me to listen. "Can't you hear the neighbors talking?" I am shocked. My mom is a bright and rational woman. I point out that she can't hear through the walls of two houses, and she doesn't seem to get it.

I speak to my brothers and sister about this problem, but they don't think it is serious. I visit with mom often and hear more and more that bothers me. She insists that the neighbors told her that my deceased father will be here soon. She continues to think that she can hear the neighbors talking inside their house. She believes that they talk about her all the time. My sister begins to agree with me that mom has a problem, but I don't get too far with my brothers.

Late one night, mom walks to the neighbors and awakens them. The neighbor angrily calls my brother who is a physician. My brother makes mom an appointment to see a doctor to get medication for her hallucinations.

This whole issue of taking care of mom is overwhelming. I have called her almost every day since my dad died in 1992. She tells me that I was her lifeline during that lonely time. She says, "Jan, I don't know what I would have done without you."

Her sadness hurts my heart.

I think she has been grieving for dad for the last twelve years. Now, she is afraid she may have to grieve for a daughter. I am worried that she is choosing to go first.

I don't feel obligated to call her every day. I want to talk to her. My mom lived her life through my dad. They were crazy about each other. I grew up in a Leave-It-To-Beaver family. My dad would want me to check on her for him.

Mom's problems continue. She isn't taking good care of herself or eating enough. I call my sister and brothers and say that we need to get together and talk to mom. Either we need to hire someone to spend part of the day and cook and clean for her, or she needs to go into assisted living. Everyone arrives at Mom's for lunch.

She knows her status quo is threatened. She sits in her favorite chair and looks at us with defiant and frightened eyes. Her voice agrees to have help but her rigid body signals her anguish.

She knows the jig is up.

On a friend's recommendation, I call Home Sweet Home. Mom isn't too friendly at first but soon warms up to Virginia, her new helper. Physically, she doesn't respond as well as we hoped she would. She won't eat and begins to stay in bed all the time.

Bill and I go to see her on Mother's Day, and I fix her a special lunch. She gets out of bed to eat but soon is lying down on the sofa. I sit beside her and talk to her. I ask her questions about her childhood. She tells me stories about Gracie, her collie, and her tree house.

I fear that I will lose her soon. She is slipping from us. It is her choice. My problem with blood clots continues along with my mother's problems. Because of all these clots, I spend an inordinate amount of time in the ultrasound department of the Smith-Glynn-Calloway Clinic in Springfield. Joann and Sandy are the techs in that clinic. We bond immediately. We talk about our families and books as well as the condition of my legs. They don't want me to be sick. The best way I can describe them is to quote from Anne Lamott's book Bird by Bird. She writes, "A big heart is both a clunky and delicate thing; it doesn't protect itself and it doesn't hide. It stands out like a baby's fontanel, where you can see the pulse through." These women let their big hearts shine as they work with me.

Dr. Goodwin puts me back in the hospital. As I am sitting on my bed in St. John's in May, an array of yellow, orange, purple, and white blossoms reigns on my bedside table. The card reads, " Love, Joann and Sandy."

I smell their souls in its fragrance. These women and their flowers are a gift.

That very week, my brother checks my mom into a different hospital. I am not allowed to leave my bed. I feel hollow inside. I want to see her, to tell her I love her.

I call her on the phone, but she isn't responding well. My sadness is multiplied when Dr. Goodwin says that I should not go to Columbia to Daniel's law school graduation. I cannot stop crying. This illness is keeping me from two people that I love so much.

Bill skips the graduation and stays with me. A scan finds another tumor. The cancer is back in all its ugly glory.

Our son Matt flies in from Colorado. He goes to Columbia with Daniel for the graduation. He films every minute of it so that I can be there, too. These gifts of loving keep coming when I need them the most.

After a week, I get out of the hospital, but Mom does not. She is transferred to Cox North where my brother practices. Bill and I go to see her every day.

My leg is swollen, and I walk with a limp. Mom is barely able to talk but seems to recognize us until her last few days.

I put on some Toujours Moi perfume on Saturday. It was my grandmother's favorite. I sit on the bed next to Mom so that her mother's familiar scent will take her from this world to the next. I lean close and breathe in my mom's own comforting smell, whisper that I love her, and tell her that it's okay for her to go. "Dad is waiting for you." I kiss her on the forehead one last time.

Chapter Twenty-Five

My brothers, sister, and I sit down at a table at the funeral home. The first question asked is if the casket will be open or closed. I answer "Closed" at the same time that another voice says, "Open." I say that a closed casket was Mom's only request to me about her service. I have to honor her wish. Dissension swirls around us. Voices rise in anger and dismay when only our sorrow should show its face.

I feel raw as if my skin and emotions are being scraped off by a potato peeler, layer by layer. Working in tandem, cancer and grief are stripping me down to my most vulnerable self.

Grief gives my sister, brothers, and me a royal punch in the gut. Who can explain how any of us acts? Perhaps there is no right or wrong; there is simply sorrow.

I can feel my parents' tears as if they were sitting beside me.

I am exhausted. My emotions are swollen in my head, and they seem to run into the fatness of my leg. It throbs, as does my heart.

We meet with the preacher to discuss the memorial service. I ask him to pray for us as we are having trouble dealing with all this. After the meeting, I hug my sister and brother. "Let's quit arguing and do this the way Mom and Dad would want us to. I can't take any more of this." We stand in a tight circle and weep.

I have my first chemo the next day. I'm sitting in the recliner in that miserable room when my phone rings. Gail says that we have a meeting with the preacher who will actually perform the service. The meeting will be while I'm in the chemo chair. I don't care anymore. I tell Gail to represent us both. She says that she will.

Gail is now upset and worried about me. Bill is angry and trying to protect me while grieving for my mom. I am grieving the loss of my mom and the loss of my freedom to the sting of the IV.

This is the week from hell.

Chapter Twenty-Six

The comfort of faith – do I ever need it now! It is critical to my healing. From the moment I was diagnosed, I have seen the power of love from the community of faith that I know from living in Kimberling City for thirty-one years. That community is not just the United Methodist Church that we attend. I receive bags of cards from people all over Stone County. I am on the prayer list of more churches than I knew existed and in the personal prayers of so many people.

A couple stops me at Wal-Mart to give me a hug. They say that they pray for me every morning. I am humbled by their goodness. I don't want to let them or anyone else down. Cancer touches so many families, leaving sadness and destruction in its wake. We need hope that this illness is beatable. As long as I'm alive, I give hope to someone else. That is important to me.

It takes a village to raise a child and a community to beat this illness. Feeling the power of others' prayers makes me strong in my soul. A fellow church-goer stops me in the street to ask how I am. The grocery store checker hugs me and says I look great. I feel their kindness and compassion. I love them for it.

I belong to a book club, a yoga studio, Peace and Serenity group, a tennis group, and a retired teachers club. I talk with Shirley, a 13-year survivor of ovarian cancer. She is my mentor. I met her at the doctor's office shortly after I was diagnosed with ovarian cancer. She has called me ever since to see how I am doing. Shirley and the women in these groups encourage and inspire me. They pray for me. They may never know how much they mean to me but their spirituality lifts my soul.

Chapter Twenty-Seven

My faith, Bill, our sons and their families get me through this terrible week. Bill reads my words about my mom at her service. He begins as I wrote, "You are doing fine, sugar. I am so proud of you." The gentle rhythm and the sweet sounds of my mother's soft Southern voice are among my earliest memories. I will forever love the sound of a Southern drawl because of the way that voice touched me. Our mother's gift to her children is a legacy of love. She learned that love from her parents who had learned it from theirs. She passed it onto us—love your family with all your heart and soul. I call my granddaughter Eliza "my sugar." She argues with me and says, "No, Grandma, I'm Eliza." However, when her granddad referred to Eliza as sugar, Eliza replied, "No, Granddad, I'm Grandma's sugar."

That word sugar has come a long way from the cotton land of central Louisiana to the hills of the Ozarks to the base of the Rockies. It is a symbol of my mom's love for all of us. It's a circle that will not be broken as I send it on to my grandchildren. It is also a symbol of the love that an entire community continues to give me. They are all "sugar" in my heart.

After the memorial service, we return to Mom's house. Aunts, uncles, cousins, siblings, our children, and grandchildren are perched all over the house. I am exhausted. My sadness is expanding, as is my leg. Everyone is here who should be except my mom and dad.

I choose a spot on the sofa just as my siblings and their families enter the room. One voice demands that we begin dividing mom's possessions. I am so tired that I want to lie down on the floor, not argue about who gets what. "I'm not going to do that today. We need time to think about what each of us would like to have. I will try to set a date in about two months that will be agreeable to everyone." The rest of the voices chime in agreement. We need time, and we know it.

I remember years ago when my dad asked me to be the executor. I lived close by and was married to a lawyer. That made me the logical choice. My dad also trusted me. He said that he knew I would be fair. His words run over and over in my mind. Bill says that I am bending over backward to follow Dad's wishes. I don't want to do it any other way. I love my parents and my brothers and sister.

The experience of my mother's dying throbs throughout my body. My family feels this painful event with individual and collective waves of grief. I learn that we don't all act the same as these waves pound our defenses. I also know that nothing is as important to me as family ties, no matter how we wound one another in pain and sorrow. My mother's legacy is intact.

I am hurting on the surface and under my skin. The pain of double loss, of my body to cancer and my mom to the earth, eats into the marrow of my bones and the grace of my soul.

Each of my siblings feels grief true to his or her own nature. I feel fragile like a dandelion clinging to its stalk, sensing that a strong wind can disperse it in a second. I sit in a gale holding onto my husband's arm as sadness, jealousy, anger, and love swirl around me. I can tell no more. I cannot look at this illness from my brothers' and sister's perspectives. Their behavior is what it is, as is mine. They are my family, and I love them. As Richard Ford says in The Lay of the Land, "At some point – and its arrival may not be obvious, so you have to be on the look-out for it – you have to let life please you if it will, and consign the past to its midden."

Chapter Twenty-Eight

My sister Gail is another story. We share a tight past. I do not remember my life as a child without Gail. I never had my own room. I shared with Gail. We bathed together as small children. We gauged our worth as developing girls by the changes in each other's bodies. We weren't impressed with the results, but we continued to change together.

Gail and I are nineteen months apart. I'm the older sister. To this day, I feel protective of her. We have not lost our closeness to one another. She is concerned and caring throughout this ordeal. This isn't always easy for her. She went through a difficult divorce and needed comfort just as I do. Gail didn't have an abundance of confidence in herself when the divorce began. Mom's death and my constant battle to stay alive are difficult for her. She watches as her support system crumbles around her. I can hear the fear in her voice when she asks how I am.

Yet, Gail grows stronger every day. Her confidence creeps out as she realizes that she can take care of herself. She is dating and knows the kind of man she wants. I don't think she will settle for less. She and I talk on the phone. We share the worries and joys of our sons, their wives, and our grandchildren. I count on her support. I hope I am there for her as she is for me.

Chapter Twenty-Nine

It is a month since Mom's death, and I am back in the hospital. I am on the table again but not completely sedated. I converse with Dr. Lubisich. He looks young enough to be my son. I ask him where he went to medical school. It's a ruse for finding out if he is actually old enough to have MD behind his name. He humors me as he installs a Greenfield filter in the Vena Cava as well as three overlapping veinous stents. With my history of blood clots I could be a sitting duck, waiting for a clot to escape into my lungs. The Greenfield filter is to prevent that from happening. The stents are to clear out the veins in my legs. He also inserts a chemotherapy port in my left femoral artery. This is my second port as I had the first removed after my first round of chemo in the hope that I would never need another.

That hope ends today.

Dr. Lubisich is a gift. After my surgery, he consults with Bill about my progress. Dr. Luby, as the nurses call him, reports that I quizzed him prior to the procedure about his medical school background. When he told me that he had gone to Stanford, I replied that I had a son who had gone to Harvard. He knew that Daniel went to Rhodes. He tells Bill that he knows all about our family. I don't remember much about that conversation. I do remember that I felt comfortable with that young doctor who doesn't appear old enough to be wielding a scalpel in my body.

Gail was with Bill in the surgery waiting room. She is with me a day later as we walk the aisles of the grocery store. We run into Dr. Luby near the cashiers. "Dr. Lubisich," I yelled. He answers, "Mrs. Kirsch, how is your leg?" I pull up my pants leg in Price Cutter and flash my skinny leg. So many people have looked at my body; I have no shame or pride. I want health—that's all.

Chapter Thirty

I am enrolled in my chemo regimen again. I am getting my treatment in the Branson office now. It is small and more personable than the Springfield office. I can't believe I am stuck to an IV again.

July is almost gone but my 40th high school reunion is here. My hair and scalp feel tingly. When I brush my hair getting ready to leave the house, some of it falls out. I decide to deny the reality of the loose silver strands dancing on my black dress and pretend that isn't happening for at least this one night.

We arrive at the hotel and see former classmates at the door. I expect superficiality but immediately connect with a friend who lost his partner to cancer a few months before. I feel grief at his loss. He touches me with his concern for my battle. We cut away the chitchat and go straight to the black and white of the reality we both live. There is no reunion rah rah here. We are just two old friends sharing sadness in a noisy room filled with voices from the past.

Chapter Thirty-One

It's morning. I'm supposed to meet my siblings to divide my parents' belongings. I wake up nauseous, throwing up repeatedly.

I call my mom's house. My sister-in-law answers the phone. I tell her I'm sick, but I'll be there in an hour.

"We don't have time to wait for you to get started. We have to get back home."

Dismay and chemo's havoc choke in my throat. I hang up the phone and vomit again.

She's concerned with a three and one half-hour drive home. I'm trapped on a frightening road that leads to a painful death. Yet, a kindred part of me understands. She hasn't been here. It's not her fault.

We are in two different worlds.

Bill and I arrive at mom's house an hour late. The four of us divide mom's possessions from the world we share with grace, smiles, and tears. We find forgiveness in the intricate, lacy pattern of a familiar Christmas tablecloth. It tells the stories that unite us. We are not perfect, but we are family.

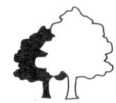

Chapter Thirty-Two

I finish three chemo treatments and have a PET scan. I call this the "God of All Scans." It is "The Decider." I call Laura, Dr. Goodwin's nurse, to get the results. She says that Dr. Goodwin will return my call. That is not good news. If the scan is clear, Laura could give me the results. I wait.

I have a tennis match tonight. I decide to forget the holy scan and play tennis as usual. I play a few games, and my cell phone rings. Dr. Goodwin is on the line. The chemo is slowing the growth of the tumor but not as quickly as he wants. He recommends that I consider other options. I don't want to turn around and face my friends. I don't want to be the one on that court who has cancer. I don't want to be sick. I tell my friends that the tumor is shrinking, but my doctor wants me to consider other options. "Let's play tennis," I say. My friends understand. They take their cue from me and try to beat my socks off. I hit that ball with all the anger I feel at my cancer. I play a heck of a game.

The women I play tennis with are steadfast in their determination that I will beat this illness. They show their faith by their decision to treat me as if nothing is wrong with me. I bask in their confidence. I forget that I am different from anyone else—playing tennis on a Wednesday night with my friends, laughing at miss-hit balls and sharing the latest gossip. I played tennis through my first chemo with a wig on my head and queasiness in my stomach. Now, I play tennis with my leg swollen with lymphedema hanging out for all the world to see from under my short tennis skirt. It slows me down, but they don't give me an inch. Their attitude is what I need. Every hour I spend on the tennis court is an hour of being normal. That is all I want—no breaks, no pity, no special treatment. I want to be a player—nothing more.

No, that isn't honest.

I want to be a winner.

Chapter Thirty-Three

Back at home in my sweaty tennis clothes, I sit down with Bill and give him the news. We decide to try radiation again. We call Dr. Rogers the next morning to get his advice. He recommends Dr. Ross McBride, the newest member of the St. John's radiation/oncology department. Dr. McBride is somewhat unconventional and open to new ideas, which is what my treatment requires. Bill and I feel better after that recommendation. We call Dr. Goodwin and tell him that I want to see Dr. McBride. His office makes the appointment for us.

Chapter Thirty-Four

We walk into the waiting room for Dr. McBride's office. Peaches-and-cream Lynn is behind the desk. A smile lights her face as she welcomes me back. Neither of us wants me to be there again. However, this is better than chemo. I take solace in that.

Dr. McBride's nurse Kathy calls us back to his office. I go through the routine— weight, blood pressure, and questions about pain. "On a scale of one to ten, how do you rate your pain?" I would love never to hear that question again or see the smiley faces that accompany that question on the chart on the wall. Heaven may be never having to go into a doctor's office or hospital again. There is a quote by Albert Camus that I keep in my mind whenever I enter a waiting room. "Even in the midst of winter, I knew there lay wihin me an invincible summer." Cancer is winter in my body, but somehow I reach down in my soul and find summer there. I use it to warm the cold of winter. It is my secret talisman in this battle for my life.

Dr. McBride is a balding man in his forties. He is a doctor who offers possibility. He is determined to help me. He and Bill talk about the radiation treatment. He is excited as he explains it to us. He says that he doesn't have many patients who understand the technical aspects of treatment. Bill does, and Dr. McBride enjoys Bill's intellect. Hope surrounds us all.

Chapter Thirty-Five

I hit the road to Springfield Monday morning. I live 45 miles from the radiation clinic. I go Monday through Friday for six weeks. I arrive at the clinic, wait until my name is called, and go back for treatment. The technicians smile, and I feel that warmth. I pull my pants partway down and lie on a table under a huge machine. Prior to the first treatment, my body was marked with tiny spots. They show the techs where to position me on the table. They spend as much time as they need to get my body in the right position. They leave the room, and treatment begins. I lie on the table and look up at the ceiling. There are some red lights above me. They form a cross. I pray under that cross the whole time I lie there. I pray for healing. I lie absolutely still for 10 minutes. I try my yoga breathing techniques. They help me relax.

I hear Dr. McBride's scolding voice. "Mrs. Kirsch, you must not move. You must breathe normally." The young brunette tech comes through the door. "Do you take yoga?" "Yes." "I thought so. No yoga breathing here."

I have no more problems. I save yoga breathing for home. The machine turns and hums. It makes a special sound when it delivers the radiation. I learn to count how long each delivery takes. I'm in charge of something. I know when the treatment will end.

The large, heavy metal door creaks open. The techs enter and help me off the table. We talk about their families and mine. I feel like a person with them. I concentrate on that. If I let myself think about being sealed in a room with radiation that could harm as well as help, I cannot do it. The chemo bags on the IV read hazardous, as does the writing on the radiation door. Every cancer patient knows the feeling of being alone in your body with that powerful, scary stuff seeping into it. Everyone else clears out, but the patient can't. I learn courage from this beast—courage I didn't know I have.

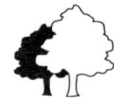

Chapter Thirty-Six

I first heard about courage in my dad's bedtime stories. He loved to tell fairy tales or stories from Greek and Norse mythology. I identified with the princesses and goddesses but wondered about the princes and gods who fought the dragons and demons. Would I be brave if I ever met a dragon?

My first dragon was going to school. I cried every day as I sat in my chair in Wilson Elementary in Little Rock, Arkansas. My teacher, Mrs. Kinney, tried to make me feel comfortable. She called me at home and came by to see me. I did well academically, but the tears still came.

My dad decided to get into the act. He began telling me stories of Janet the Giant Killer. She visited him at his office during the day. She was brave and bold. She slew dragons regularly. I stopped crying at school. In the man's world of the fifties, my dad gave me the gift of power. I could be strong and be a girl.

My dad died before I was diagnosed with cancer. He was my hero. He left me Janet the Giant Killer. She rises up to slay the dragon time and again. It comes in the guise of a spot on a PET scan, but it is there. So is she.

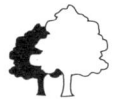

Chapter Thirty-Seven

Bill and I are members of the United Methodist Church in Kimberling City, Missouri. We attend Sunday School almost every Sunday. We feel close to the members of this class. It is unique because people say whatever they think, believe or doubt. We share our vulnerability about our faith, concerns about the church's silent voice as war rages in Iraq, and the continuing issue of segregation in church pews. We tackle the tough issues, the put-your-money-where-your-mouth-is issues, that show whether our Christianity is just talkin' or is doing the walkin.' At least for that hour, we all suspend judgment and try to accept one another as we are.

Our teacher is Martha Bohner. She used to be the editor of the Branson Daily News and now works in public relations for Silver Dollar City. Martha is an intelligent woman with an abundance of faith. She accepts all the questioning in our class and turns it back around to faith. I once described our class to a member of a large fundamental church. She looked wistful as she told me that she would love to attend a class like that. She had questions but could not ask them in her church.

I can't imagine a class without questions. Our son Matt had a science teacher in junior high who didn't allow questions in class. We went to school about that one. I can't accept all I am told without thinking for myself. I don't always like what I learn, but I know more than before I asked. This is honest religion. You show your vulnerability, but you gain strength and faith.

I share my trials with cancer with this class. I feel a closeness to these people. They want the best for me. That is one of the gifts of this illness. I sense the warmth in other people's hearts. It flows to my heart and brings me joy.

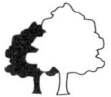

Chapter Thirty-Eight

My friend Luann has that same warmth in her heart. She has big green eyes and a great laugh. She was my partner in the great mushroom hair adventure. Thirty years tells of our friendship—raising our children together as we talk about everything. My boys learned about playing house from her daughter Melanie. And, Mel learned to throw a football and shoot a basket from them.

Luann taught kindergarten, and I taught high school, so we discussed kids from five to eighteen. No subject was taboo, from religion to books to shoes to hair—always our hair. My cancer diagnosis was the first thing I kept from Luann. We were supposed to be in San Diego at Melanie's wedding when I found out I had to have surgery. We already had our tickets. Daniel was going to escort Luann down the aisle. He stayed with his Dad and me instead of going to the wedding. After the surgery, I told Bill not to call Luann. I didn't want to spoil Luann's joy on Melanie's wedding day.

From the moment Luann got home from the wedding, she fought this illness with me. She sat on the front porch with me the first time I wore my wig. We shared our tears. Packages arrived from Land's End with winter caps for that bald winter. She took me to lunch and a Christmas Parade of Homes. I was so queasy we only saw two homes. She said she didn't care.

Luann and I still talk about how I don't want to die and leave Bill. She listens to my fears of not seeing Eliza and Kai grow up or never knowing Daniel's children. She listens to it all and never loses her smile. She lets her love sit right on her sleeves and comforts me. Luann Barr is a good woman. I thank God that she shares the Earth with me.

Mary Helen Short is my friend at the Kimberling Area Library. She is a ball of fire and has taken me under her wing. She and her husband Bill have decided to pray me to wellness. Once Mary Helen decides to do something, you better step out of her way. She grew up in and still talks Texas. I better get well or have a darn good reason why not. Cancer is no excuse. This pint-sized woman keeps me positive. She makes me laugh.

Bill and I attend a local charity fundraiser where we are surrounded by friends. I smile as a former student gives me a hug. She brushes a hair off my face. "Isn't it funny, Mrs. Kirsch, you took care of me in high school and now I'm taking care of you." Tears brim over, but they are a rainfall of gentle love.

Cancer makes me think about friendship and what it means. Since this illness began, I have reconnected with several old friends. Two of them live in California. Mary Lee Short lives in San Francisco with her attorney husband Randy. She was my pledge mom in the Alpha Delta Pi sorority at the University of Missouri. She and Randy live the cultured city life while Bill and I are the country cousins. She surprises me with a generous donation to the Helen Jaffe Ovarian Cancer Research Fund at the University of San Francisco. My heart swells at this unexpected gift.

My second California friend is Patti Dusel. She and I became friends in sixth grade. Patti glows with faith. You can touch it off her smile. She is a breast cancer survivor. We e-mail, talk on the phone, and get together with our husbands for dinner when they come to Missouri. I never hear Patti say one bad thing about anyone. She must hide in the closet and sound off. No one can be that sweet, but she is. Her kindness is infectious, and her support is laced with memories. My life is intertwined with hers. I want her wellness as she wants mine.

Chapter Thirty-Nine

I complete my third round of radiation. Bill always schedules a trip as a reward after I finish a regimen. My surgeon, Dr. Bonebrake, told me once, "Make hay while the sun shines." That is one piece of advice we took without question. We load the car and take off for Galveston, Texas. We spend a day exploring the city. Our cruise ship arrives, and we board for the Panama Canal.

This is my first cruise. It took me 36 years to convince Bill to take me on a cruise. He cruised for three years in the US Navy during the Vietnam War. He and I don't think of cruising in the same way! He got so seasick every time the ship went to sea that he became champion of the barf-o-rama contests. He was designated a professional by the sailors and not allowed to compete in their amateur competitions. It was a gift to me for him to go to sea again.

We eat dinner with two other couples. Twyla and Roe are from Texas while Allison and Steve are from England. To me, they both speak foreign languages! We muddle along at first but get better with each meal. Twyla is in her 70's, imposing and blond. She leans across the table and confides loudly to me in her large Texas drawl. "I can't understand a word they are saying." I know Allison and Steve are thinking the same thing. They are stuck with Texans and southern Missouri hillbillies. We can both do a number on the English language. We do share common ground in the interest we take in one another. I always look now for that common ground that we as humans share. It stands out more starkly than it did before.

We enjoy the cruise. Bill has few problems on the Celebrity Princess. She glides over the ocean. She is a big momma compared to the small gasoline tanker that he helped command in the Navy.

The Panama Canal is a wonder, but the poverty we see in countries such as Jamaica is not. I look at the world through the eyes of a short-timer now. I see that poverty and know I have too much stuff. It won't go with me, so why do I think I need it? Why do I need the expensive leather purse when I see people who need to eat? How do I balance enjoying the rest of my life, leaving some wealth for our children, and helping other human beings? I don't know the answer. Yet, at night when I lie in bed and think about my mortality, I do know the answer.

I don't give enough.

Chapter Forty

I introduce Bill to the Deep South by way of our trailer travels. I was born in Alexandria, Louisiana. My mother was raised across the Red River in Pineville. My memories are filled with soft Southern voices, sweet tea and overwhelming love. The South has a special place in my heart.

We tow our trailer to the Mississippi Gulf Coast. We park it in Buccaneer Bay State Park. It is across the road from the ocean and down the road from Bay Saint Louis. Pass Christian sits on the bay around the corner. These two small towns exude the slow, casual lifestyle of the South. Tourism has not yet ruined them. There are no high-rise hotels to bow down to the rich and sacrifice their beaches to their wealthy guests. The sea and sand belong to everyone.

We buy the catch of the day at the pier as the fishing boats come in from their work. I can eat fried green tomatoes any time I want—well, any time I decide to go off my diet. We shop in the local organic store across from the waterfront. We ride our bikes from the state park into Bay Saint Louis so Bill can eat po' boys in a quaint local restaurant.

Our next stop is Mary Moseley's bright blue cottage. She is a tiny, bright-eyed octogenarian. The primitive images of her paintings bring to mind Grandma Moses. We buy two of her boldly bright images to bring Mississippi into our Missouri home.

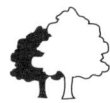

Chapter Forty-One

One of the wonders of Bay Saint Louis is Saint Rose de Lima Catholic Church. Bill and I get up on Sunday and dress for church. I put on a long gray-ribbed dress and backless black heeled sandals. I hang silver hoops from my ears and my wrists; Bill wears a short sleeve white cotton shirt, beige slacks and loafers without socks.

Picture intense blue skies above a small white frame church with a wooden cross stationed in the front. Both black and white people enter with curly haired babies in their arms, irreverent teenagers, and slow-stepping grandparents by their sides. The church is packed when we get inside. We sit at the end of a pew and have to look around a powerful wooden beam in order to see the priest and choir at the front of the sanctuary. Father Sebastian is from the Caribbean. He is short, dark-haired, and handsome. He preaches in lilting, musical English that carries traces of the island he calls home.

But the faith of this place spills out in its music. The choir leader presides at the piano with majestic joy. He raises his arm, his black hand moves, and the choir comes to life. The voices ring out with Southern black soul and faith. They move me. I feel stirrings from my early childhood. I have heard those voices before, singing in the river baptizing and praising God.

The song that touches me most is "Down by the Riverside." It brings me to tears. They follow that song with "Just As I Am." That one stirs my heart also. These are songs of my childhood. I can hear my daddy's and Granddad Jones' voices in my ear. They remind me of where I come from. We are all a part of our past even as we make our future. After almost two hours, the service is over. I have DONE BEEN to church this morning!

Chapter Forty-Two

We go back another Sunday. It is confirmation day for about 12 children. All but two are black and seem to range in age from around 8 to about 12. The boys stand tall in white shirts and the girls in white dresses. The choir sings out, "Daniel, Daniel, are you ready to serve the Lord?" Young Daniel takes the mike and sings, "Yes, Lord, yes." Every child answers in song. I feel music in my heart when I leave that church. It reminds me of a verse from Proverbs, "A cheerful heart is good medicine but a crushed spirit dries up the bones." That church helps me heal. I have no space in my body for dried up bones.

Chapter Forty-Three

Faith is an important part of my life because it gives me hope. In *Heretics*, G. K. Chesterton said, "Hope is the power of being cheerful in circumstances that we know are desperate." That sums up how I feel with the ovarian cancer diagnosis. This is the fourth most deadly of all cancers. When I read the statistics, fear grips my soul. My older son Matt has a rational approach to life. He hides his emotions behind his reason. However, after my diagnosis, he was the first to say, "Mom, you are not a statistic." I felt hope. It comes again by way of an Episcopal church in Bay Saint Louis.

The healing service sign on the church is like a beacon. My heart hammers as we approach the drive. The ocean skips in and out at my back as Bill parks the truck. We step out onto the gravel driveway. The white Episcopal church and its rainbow-colored stained glass windows sparkle under the brilliant blue of the sky. I want to be here. I don't like the fake fanatical healing service of a Benny Hinn, but I sense this will be different.

About a dozen people are in the church. They are all women except for Bill. An older lady with short white hair and a face full of pain sits in a pew near the front. She is soon joined by a plump young woman of about 18 and a mannish woman who looks to be in her 60's.

Bill and I are in the pew behind them on the left side of the church. He is wearing a white shirt, purple shorts, and tennis shoes. I am dressed in black linen slacks with a beige tee-shirt under a long-sleeved beige linen shirt. The rest of the congregation sits behind us.

The brilliantly hued stained glass windows leap out at us from the pristine white walls. The woman priest and her white-haired assistant enter in pure white robes. The priest is 35 to 40 with thick unruly brown hair escaping from a bushy ponytail. She wears an elaborately printed shawl over her robe.

The priest greets us, and we use the Prayer Book for the Healing Service. We kneel at the altar. The young priest asks me, "Who do you need prayers for?"

"Myself and a friend's son."

Her hands rest on my head as she prays for healing. She anoints my forehead with oil while marking it with the sign of the cross. Again, her hand finds my head, and she prays quietly.

I feel peace.

Chapter Forty-Four

We return home and go to our church on Sunday. "God never gives you more than you can handle." The well-meaning woman pats my hand and smiles at me.

I want to scream. "Oh, well, he just overdosed me."

I hate that remark and that philosophy. I detest it because it assumes that God gives me cancer. It carries a sanctimonious punch to the gut. I can hear the woman's thoughts. "God must have given cancer to you for something you did wrong. I, however, don't have it."

One of our pastors touches my hand as I walk by him. "How are you doing?" "Fine," I say. He looks at me closely. "How are you really doing?" I have the sense that he almost hopes that I will fall apart in front of him; that I will confess that I am actually awful.

Cancer is difficult for all of us. If we do not have it, we feel so grateful that we don't. When we look at someone who does, a part of us is so glad that it is him or her and not us. Guilt overwhelms us. I know this because I felt this before I had cancer. It helps me deal with the comments that hurt. In a strange way, I feel compassion for the struggling onlooker. A woman told me once to get well because if I didn't, a lot of women would be waiting to go after my husband. I didn't know what to say. I wanted to cry.

She meant to encourage me to get well. I forgive her. I am no saint. I reek of the sins I hear the preacher denounce—jealousy, selfishness, giving too little. Cancer doesn't take away my faults. It sets them in bold print for me to see. I don't want to share Bill with any other woman. I fight to be with him. I won't give him up without a battle.

Chapter Forty-Five

Bill is my lover and my friend. We met at the University of Missouri. He whitewashed my eye when we were supposed to be whitewashing the big M at one end of the football stadium. I had to go to the university clinic and walk back to the sorority house with a huge bandage over my eye.

I had a date that night. When the buzzer beeped my code, I went down to the living room. It wasn't my date. It was Bill. He said, "I thought we could have a blind date tonight." I was mad and crazy about this guy at the same time. "I don't need a blind date. I already have a date." I sent him packing.

My fury didn't last long. We had a date the next weekend. We celebrated our 37th wedding anniversary this year. I don't regret my choice. Bill's health affected our marriage long before mine did. He was diagnosed with Type I juvenile diabetes six years after we married. That was a struggle. When Bill was diagnosed, I knew almost nothing about diabetes. The first time he became furious about nothing, I could not believe it. Low blood sugar turns Dr. Jekyl into Mr. Hyde. I learned to get him a glass of orange juice and forget what he said when his sugar was low. If it happened in the middle of the night, I called Matt or Daniel. They could reason with him when I couldn't.

I learned to fix healthy foods and always carry snacks. I recognized the signs of low blood sugar before Bill did. If he looked pale, began to move slowly or sweated for no reason, then I knew he needed to eat.

Before my last PET scan, we ran into a woman whose husband died of lung cancer. When I left the room, she spoke to Bill about being a caregiver. She talked to Bill about taking care of himself. Bill didn't remind her that I was his caregiver. I resented that.

I don't like being the one who is always ill.

I was miffed that he didn't tell her that I take care of him. If I am honest, I don't want to be the only one with a problem. I don't like to feel weak. I want to be energetic and vital. I don't want Bill to leave me behind in the race for health. I do want Bill to take care of himself. I want him to remember that he is not the only caregiver in the family. I have been one for 31 years. I don't know if I have been as good to Bill as he is to me. I can't consider life without him.

Chapter Forty-Six

The skeletal trees of a Missouri January pass my window as our truck moves down the road towards Gulf Shores, Alabama. We play tennis, hike and walk the beach and then switch our base to Destin, Florida. We sign up to play tennis one morning with the seniors in Fort Walton Beach. A ninety-year-old man joins me on the court. He is tall and wiry and doesn't move except to raise his arm to swing at a ball. I think to myself, "I guess when they say senior tennis they mean senior tennis."

We are way behind when he says to me, "I'm no good anymore. I guess I should hang up my racket."

"Oh, no," I answer. "I'll play a little harder." I kill myself going after every ball. We win. The grin on his wrinkled face is my reward. "You're not only cute but you can play tennis, too."

As Bill and I walk off our courts I tell him the story. "It's a nice compliment, but I don't think he can actually see what I look like."

Chapter Forty-Seven

We travel on to Amelia Island. I reconnect with a friend I haven't seen in 20 years. We were with her at the death of her fiancée. We are her youngest son's godparents.

Kathy and I spend a morning sharing coffee, memories and realities of the present. She tells me that it is worth the drive to go to Plains, Georgia, to attend Jimmy Carter's Sunday School class. We decide to make the trip.

Jimmy Carter is a humble man. I am talking about a former president— the most powerful man in the world for four years. We go through minimum security to sit in a pew in a simple Baptist church and learn from this intelligent man. Before he enters, a woman from the congregation tells us how to behave. We are told not to stand or clap as he enters the room. We are not to address him as Mr. President. These are Jimmy Carter's instructions. For this hour, he is our Sunday School teacher.

He teaches the regular Bible lesson. It deals with treating other human beings as you would your family. He calls on people in the audience and expects a reply. There is no sleeping in this class.

Neither is there any mistake about the faith of this man. He practices what he preaches. He lives in a comfortable ranch house in town. That home has no visible trappings of greatness.

Jimmy Carter is highly involved with Habitat for Humanity. He has helped build thousands of homes. He flew in from Palestine last night. He helped oversee elections there. He plans to leave for Geneva this afternoon to meet with Condoleezza Rice and the Secretary General of the United Nations to talk with them about his concern about the elections. After the lesson, he and Rosalyn stand at the front of the church for as long as it takes for everyone to have their photo made with them.

This man breathes humility. He is accountable for the way he walks the earth. His life makes a difference.

He makes a difference for me. He shows me the great strength of humility in a world overwhelmed with pride and power. He finishes the lesson that cancer began. It doesn't matter who you are; it's how you respond that matters. If nothing else, I can leave this legacy to our sons.

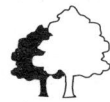

Chapter Forty-Eight

We leave Plains and drive to Slidell, Louisiana. We meet 10 members of our church at the Methodist Relief Headquarters. We spend a week helping families rebuild their homes after Hurricane Katrina. The devastation touches my very bones. It makes me ache to see it. We didn't expect to see this ruin and decay in the United States of America.

Our team is helping a single woman drywall her house. In the midst of that work, her mother dies. We help another woman redo her ceiling and find out that the roof is rotten. Her husband is dying of cancer. A third woman's yard is piled so high with debris that we can't see the ground when we arrive. She weeps when she sees how much we did in one day while she was at work. The fourth family we meet lost 17 trees in the storm. They live in a FEMA trailer. Their home is uninhabitable. They help us clean out muck and ruined belongings from their home.

We are here six months after the hurricane. I ask the mother, "Who is helping you?" She said, "The only people who have helped us are God's people."

Christians talk a lot about being good people and going to church. I am skeptical about so much talk. I felt better about us as a group after I listened to that mother. We did what faith says that we should do. We did help our neighbors.

These people make a difference in my life. They survived a catastrophe and didn't quit. I respect them. I won't quit fighting my disaster. I want my family to respect me.

I want to respect myself.

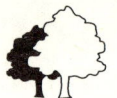

Chapter Forty-Nine

Bill and I raised two sons. Matthew was our first. He came into our lives in the midst of the Vietnam War. I found out that I was pregnant a few months before Bill's ship deployed to Vietnam. Matt was three weeks old when Bill returned.

I spent the last few months of my pregnancy with my parents. They took me to the hospital when it was time for Matt to be born. I missed his dad. I felt like I had this baby all alone. When I first heard him cry, he was sealed in my heart forever. I would protect him no matter what.

Matt is 35 today. He has Harvard undergraduate and Duke law diplomas hanging on his walls. He is an Assistant United States Attorney in Denver. Matt has won awards all his life, but they have never turned his head. When he was recognized as the youngest inductee of his high school's Sports Hall of Fame, he praised another young man who played tennis before him. He is a good man who does what is right. When speaking about his dad at Bill's retirement, he said that what he and his brother remember most about their dad is that Bill always taught them to do the right thing. Matt learned his lesson well. He is the son any mother would claim. I am unabashedly proud of him.

Matt didn't cry when I told him about my cancer. He said that I would beat it. His wife Kerri tells me that my illness doesn't seem to faze him. She is concerned about him. He goes to work as if nothing unusual has happened.

I am stunned. Doesn't Matt care about my illness? I flash on memories of Matt as a child and a young man. My reflections freeze and turn into icy sadness.

I cannot live with the coldness. I call Matt and tell him what Kerri had said. "Mom, it hits me at the strangest times. I was sitting at my desk at work and felt tears on my face. I never know when it will happen."

I know selfishness and joy at the same instant. I am glad and sad that he feels sorrow. As a mom, I don't want to bring him sadness. As a human, I need to know his pain. At my most wounded, I need to know his love.

Our second son Daniel was born while Bill was in law school and I was in graduate school in education. Bill wanted to watch the birth, but my older doctor didn't allow fathers in the room. Bill watched from a window. The doctor saw him. His face mottled with red, and his voice filled with anger. I was afraid for my baby. I felt animalistic about protecting him. I was torn but waved Bill away from the window. I would do whatever it took to save that baby.

I held Daniel one night when he woke to nurse. I thought how much I loved him. I knew I would remember that feeling forever. I do remember that moment in the silent house with only the furnace kicking on and off for melody. I will love him forever.

Daniel is 33 now. He has Rhodes College undergraduate and University of Missouri Law School degrees in his office. He is in private practice but looking for a job in public service. Daniel has the gifts of compassion and respect for his fellow man. These gifts were evident as a third grader when he refused to wear his nice school clothes to school. When I scolded him for wearing holey play clothes he replied, "Mom, my friend Andy only has holey clothes. He will feel bad if I wear nice clothes." "Wear whatever you'd like, Daniel." I was awed by his unreserved empathy. Today, I recognize his strength of soul and love him for his goodness. As with his brother, any mother would claim him, and I am unabashedly proud of him.

I have felt his closeness throughout my ordeal. He was with Bill when I came out of that first surgery. He wept with his father at the doctor's words. Daniel decided to go to law school at the University of Missouri instead of Tennessee. I think he made that decision to be close to us when we needed him. I will not forget that gift.

Daniel and his wife may leave Missouri to find the job he wants. I struggle with that idea and want to keep them close. I suggest all the reasons they should stay in Missouri. I almost convince myself that it is best for them.

I feel desperate. I know the cancer influences me. I am afraid I will not live as long as I would like. I am afraid I will not get to see them as much as I want. I am afraid that I will never know Daniel's children; that I will be a face in a picture frame by the time they arrive.

I lie awake at night and see Daniel again as that tiny baby. I lay that fear on my blanket and let it go. I want what is best for him. I set us both free from my fear. He has my blessing, and he knows it.

Chapter Fifty

Bill and I come home after the week in Slidell. We enjoy three months of freedom. That ends with my PET scan in May. The cancer is back. I feel sick to my stomach. How many more times will I hear Dr. Goodwin say, "You have a recurrence."

I want to slap him, slap the world, break the PET machine. I replay the scene with Dr. Goodwin saying, "You are fine." Reality always breaks through and spoils the dream.

Dr. Goodwin suggests we try chemo for the third time. He doesn't think I will lose my hair with this chemo.

I dread the first treatment. I sit down in that chair and want to scream. But I don't. I let them fill me with those questionable chemicals again. Two weeks after the first treatment, I notice my hair is shedding. I pretend it is nothing.

I can't face baldness again.

I endure three treatments and have a CAT scan. The tumor is slowly shrinking but not enough. Dr. Goodwin recommends we try radiation again. In a crazy way, I rejoice. I detest chemo and won't have to go through it again. We make an appointment with Dr. McBride at the radiation/oncology center.

Dr. McBride discusses the possibility of trying the Cyberknife. Bill and I talked about this option before we met with him. We hoped that he would suggest it. The Cyberknife is new to the Springfield area. The doctors have not yet tried it on a case of ovarian cancer. I agree to become the first. There are no guarantees.

The beauty of the Cyberknife is that the machine delivers an extremely potent dose of radiation to a very defined area. It does the most possible damage to the tumor without damaging surrounding tissue or organs. I am ready to try it.

The doctors saw two spots of cancer that they intend to treat with the Cyberknife. One of those spots is in a difficult place to reach. In order to help them find that spot accurately during the treatment, four gold seeds have to be implanted in my body as locators. As with any hospital procedure, I have to go several days early to give blood for testing and to answer questions about my health, living will, etc.

I hate to walk through that tall glass door. It means pain and fear every time I enter. It is a gigantic reminder that all is not well in my body.

A brown-haired woman doctor I have never met does the laparoscopic implantation procedure. She is serious and sad when she speaks to me. I want to reassure her that I will be fine. I want to tell her that her somber attitude doesn't help me, her patient.

I want to scream.

Instead, I lie on the table and do what she asks. I keep my thoughts on the hope of the Cyberknife.

Chapter Fifty-One

Next, I meet with the technicians who work with the Cyberknife. They are the same technicians who helped me during my previous radiation treatments. It is old home week when I arrive for the first appointment. Kristi, Becky and Tim make me feel like a princess. Their desire for my healing permeates their professionalism. I can hear it in their voices. These are good solid people. I'm glad they are taking care of me. I have confidence in them.

I lie on a plastic-like material on the treatment table. Kristi, Becky and Tim mold the white material to my body. Since I am worried about my leg swelling during the treatment, they elevate it for me. After the mold is complete, both the mold and I are sent to the hospital for a PET scan.

I am also issued a special vest for this treatment. It is futuristic black with white stripes and a skin-tight fit. It has cords hanging from it. These will be attached to the Cyberknife so that it can adjust its delivery of radiation to my breathing.

I feel like I stepped in from Star Wars. So do a few of the hospital personnel. They do double takes when they see me. I feel proud of myself—like a pioneer. I tell the nurse that I was a polio pioneer in 1954. I was one of the first children in the nation to get the live polio vaccine. My school in Little Rock was a test school. I have the pin to prove it.

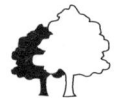

Chapter Fifty-Two

The young woman who takes blood samples ushers me into the waiting room behind the waiting room. I love these hospitals. It is always hurry up and wait and wait some more. I tell her that my veins are tiny and abused by chemotherapy. I tell her that my right arm is better than my left to stick. I tell her to warm the vein first and it will cooperate. She looks at the veins in my left arm and says that she will try that one. She doesn't warm the vein. She sticks me twice with no success other than blowing the vein. I say, "So, what are you going to do now?" She says, "Get help."

The nurse enters and asks what the problem is. I tell her the young woman didn't use the arm I suggested or warm the vein. The nurse shakes her head. "I always listen to the patient." Inside I think, maybe you should teach that to the techs. Outwardly, I say thank you and breathe a sigh of relief when she brings in a warm pad for the vein in my right arm.

A small wiry bespectacled tech enters the room next. He consults his clipboard and starts asking me questions. How many surgeries have I had? What kind of surgeries? I reply, "To begin with, a radical hysterectomy." "Which breast did they take?" he asks.

My confidence blasts out the door. "That would be neither," I answer. I look at Bill with disbelief. The tech continues to the next question without missing a breath. I do not feel safe with this man. Bill asks him about the procedure. He says that I will have a CAT scan and a PET scan in two different rooms. Bill questions that and says that he understood that I would have them both done on the same machine. The tech doesn't agree. He injects me with the dye for the test and leaves the room.

Once the dye is injected, I am supposed to rest for about 45 minutes to get the most accurate test results. I am not ready to test. I tell Bill, "I don't trust that guy. I don't want to go anywhere with him."

Bill tries to settle me down but that makes me angry. I lie there and fume. Bill gets up and leaves the room. He brings in a nurse and explains the situation. She reports that Bill is correct. I will have the tests as he thought. I tell her, "I will not go to the testing area with that tech."

She defends him as a nice man. I repeat that I will not go with him. They send someone else to get me.

Chapter Fifty-Three

I walk down the hall and lie down on my molding as instructed. The PET technicians leave the room, and the scan begins. I lie there and think about the cancer. I hope that it won't show up but know inside that it will. I listen to the machine's disembodied voice telling me what to do. I hold my breath and breathe on command. I am glad when it is over. The technicians say that they have never heard the voice on this new machine. I say that there is one problem with it. "I don't think that many hillbillies will be comfortable with the King's English. Carry on breathing is not common to the local vernacular." They laugh, and I am finished.

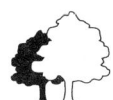

Chapter Fifty-Four

I thought I was finished. The next day, I get a call from the Cyberknife office. The technicians who ran the PET/CAT scan machine didn't run the tests properly. They need to repeat the procedure. They want to do it next week. That upsets me.

Our son Daniel is getting married in October. I want to complete the treatment and be on the road to health before that wedding. The Cyberknife nurse Karla says that she will do her best. She does, and I go back to Springfield within two days to repeat the tests. I complain to Karla about all that happened the first time. She reports it to Dr. McBride and the hospital.

I return for the tests. I'm met in the waiting room by the head of the PET scan department at St. John's Hospital. He was a student at Reeds Spring High School when I taught there. He apologizes for all that happened. He is genuine and concerned for my care. I appreciate his professionalism.

I repeat the procedure—injection, waiting, lying on the table. This time the procedure goes smoothly. I am ready for the big day on the Cyberknife table.

Chapter Fifty-Five

I arrive on a Thursday afternoon at 1:00 p.m. I wear the same clothes that I had on when the mold was made. I put on my vest. I get on the table, and the technicians and Dr. McBride fuss over my position. They leave the room and shut the door. I am alone again with the giant arm of this huge machine hovering over me. Dr. McBride and the technicians talk to me. They tell me to lie without moving until they are done. I can ask to get up if I need a break. I can listen to a favorite CD. I choose James Taylor, hoping his mellow tunes will keep me calm.

I trust these people with my life. If they don't program the machine properly, I will be in some serious hurt. I try not to think about that. I concentrate on the positive. It will work. I will be well.

A host of experts work on my treatment program. Besides Dr. McBride, there are three techs, a Cyberknife physicist, surgeon Dr. Frank Schmidt, and a nurse. Bill watches them work. The treatment on the first spot of cancer takes an hour and a half. I tune in James Taylor, and we both go to Carolina. My grandchildren fill my thoughts. Bill is ever on my mind.

I get off the table, use the restroom, and take a walk. I feel fine.

The nurse calls us back to the Cyberknife room. I get on the table again. Dr. McBride and the techs fuss over my position again. They leave the room and return again and again. They cannot get the machine to lock onto the second spot. They work for over an hour with no success. I get worried that they can't finish the job. Dr. McBride assures me they will find a solution to the problem. The Greenfield filter inside me was interfering with the Cyberknife. It will not lock into position.

In another thirty minutes, the problem is solved. I have been on the table for an hour and a half without moving, and my treatment has not started. Dr. McBride asks me if I can lie there for another hour and a half. I say, "Yes. I want to get this over with."

At about seven that evening, I get off the table. I feel queasy and throw up in the restroom. Everyone is concerned. The surgeon appears with a diet Seven-Up, the physicist with crackers. I go from nausea to a euphoric high. I am the first ovarian cancer patient in Springfield, Missouri to try this.

It is done.

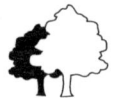

Chapter Fifty-Six

Bill and I thank everyone and hug them all. Dr. McBride walks us to our car. He tells us in the parking lot that he is leaving the hospital. He will no longer be my doctor. We don't want to hear that. We feel close to him and trust him. Our time with him is special. Sometimes, you click with someone. Bill and I heard that click with Dr. McBride. That's important when every treatment deals with life and death. Dr. McBride was another gift in the midst of my recurring nightmare.

Chapter Fifty-Seven

We drive to Daniel and Laura's wedding in Pittsburgh, Pennsylvania. We stop on the way in St. Louis at Luann and Gary Barr's house. They would meet us at the wedding in a few days. I notice my leg swelling before we leave.

The wedding is full of tears, laughter, and sheer joy but I have never seen my leg in such elephantine shape. I chose a long dress for the ceremony because I am never sure what that leg will look like. By the end of the evening, I am limping, and it hurts. I don't want the leg to interfere, so I tell no one until the night is over. The cancer or its side effects are always with me. I will not let it stop me. I recently read a quote by Ernest Hemingway: "The world breaks everyone and afterward, many are strong at the broken places."

I sometimes sense that I am forged of steel. I will be strong at my "broken places." I do not know where that comes from. I think a piece of God tears off and drops inside me. It settles inside a crack in my soul, and for a second, I see what I can be. I feel his touch and know I will fight again.

Chapter Fifty-Eight

Daniel's wife Laura is a gift I didn't expect. She and Daniel live in Springfield. I call her to chat, and she calls me. We meet for lunch. I introduce her to my yoga studio. She loves it as I do. We talk about Daniel and his search to find a meaningful job. She is Catholic, and she prays for me and my health. She loves my son above all others. I love her for that.

Laura lets me in her world and shares herself with me. She isn't threatened by how I feel about my son. She knows we are the two women in the world who love him the most.

Each of my daughters-in-law is special in her own way. I love them, regardless, because they love my sons.

Chapter Fifty-Nine

I have another PET scan. It is three months since the wedding. The scan shows that one spot has definitely shrunk, but the other is still lighting up. It has not grown but is still there. The radiation doctors recommend waiting three more months and scanning again. Bill and I are disappointed that the scan isn't clear but decide it could be worse. It could have grown.

I enjoy three more months of freedom without treatment. I have the scan again in April. There is no change. The doctors decide to wait until August and do a scan then.

Each scan costs over $2,000. I have good insurance, or we could not handle this. The Cyberknife alone was over $45,000. I have never added up the money that we or the insurance company have spent on this illness. I don't want to know. I don't want to think about it.

I throw myself into the beauty of Table Rock Lake. We water-ski and ride the Jet Ski all summer. We take picnics, books and water skis in the Ski Nautique with us. The sun on the Ozark Mountains reflects on the lake with calm and peacefulness. It seeps into my soul. I can escape here and forget. I can feel grateful. I can feel whole.

Chapter Sixty

Bill and I fly to Denver to walk in the Livestrong Challenge to raise money for cancer research. Matt, Kerri, Eliza, and Kai walk with us. I am surprised by how emotional I feel when we arrive at the stadium grounds. Bill's brother Jim and his wife Marci come from Thermopolis, Wyoming, to be there with us. Marci is armed with a camera and records the day.

Thousands of people are on the grounds. They are walking, running or biking to raise money to defeat this illness. Statistics say that one in three women and one in two men will have cancer in their lifetimes. This is a national emergency. These people are addressing that emergency with their time, their money, their energy and their hearts.

Eliza and Kai wear signs on their backs that say, "In honor of Grandma." These signs make me weep in my heart. I don't want to cry in front of these sweet, smiling faces. At the end of the walk, the survivors split from their families. We walk to the end to cheers and ringing of cowbells. I cry now. I feel the goodness of all these people I don't know.

Lance Armstrong is one of my heroes. I read his book, *It's Not About the Bike*. His words and example encourage me to fight. His contribution to cancer research is immeasurable. The walk in Denver raises $1.3 million. He sponsors similar walks in four other cities this year.

My husband wears a Livestrong yellow wristband every day. It is a reminder of his love for me and the battle the community must wage to defeat cancer. When I see that band on anyone's wrist, I feel an immediate connection. I know they are in the fight.

Chapter Sixty-One

The trials with my leg are never ending. I won't give up on ways to reduce the swelling. I try acupuncture. Jeff, the young acupuncturist, is another gift. He is warm and supportive. He believes in his craft, yet I can't tell that the acupuncture is making a difference. I need to find something else.

A tennis friend recommends a man in Springfield who practices biofeedback. I gamely call Fred Eagles at Focus on Health and make an appointment. Bill and I arrive at his office. I fill out a lengthy questionnaire about my medical history. Fred and I enter the treatment room.

I sit in a modern black leather recliner. Fred attaches bands to my head, wrists and ankles. He programs into the computer the issues I want him to treat—cancer and lymphedema. I lie back in the recliner for an hour while Fred directs the computer. On the wall, I read powerful statements from the world's great religions.

My eyes rest on the quote from Sikhism. "Be not estranged from one another for God dwells in every heart." After I was diagnosed with cancer, my eyes opened to this wisdom. I believe this. A world where this is practiced would be a different place from the one we inhabit. How could we kill other human beings if we believe this? Even in the recliner, I find myself philosophizing. I feel better when I leave.

Six months after beginning this treatment, my leg is better. It is smaller. Some days, you wouldn't notice the difference in my legs if I don't point it out to you. I am convinced this treatment works. I don't know why, but the results are good enough for me.

Bill looks at my leg and shakes his head. He calls this my hocus pocus medicine. But, he can't argue with the results. He pays for the hocus pocus with a smile on his face.

I still have to baby this leg. If I'm home, I sit on the couch and elevate the leg. If I shop all day, I pay the price. But yoga, biofeedback, diet, and exercise work to keep it under control. It's not easy.

Wednesday, I have a charity board meeting. My leg is skinny. Whoopee! I wear a short skirt and dark brown tights. For today, I have great legs (at least great for a 60-year-old woman). I take my pleasures when I can.

Chapter Sixty-Two

August 25th is here too soon. I have another PET scan. I wait several days to hear the results. I call and get the news. The scan is the same as the last time. Dr. Goodwin suggests that we request the Cyberknife tumor board to evaluate my situation again.

I go to see Dr. Bonebrake and have a pelvic exam. He can feel nothing but scar tissue. He recommends that we wait four more months and see what happens. He calls Dr. Schmidt with the Cyberknife and confers with him.

In the meantime, I am finally assigned to a new radiation/oncology doctor. Her name is Dr. Kim. She will take my case to the tumor board. I have never met this physician. I have this crazy idea that I am not just a name on a patient file. I think it matters if the doctor takes a look at me. I want her to see the live person connected to those words on a page.

I stop by the Cyberknife clinic and ask to meet her. I wait about fifteen minutes, and she steps into the waiting room. I take her hand and say, "I wanted to meet you. My life is in your hands."

Dr. Kim looks at me and says, "You're beautiful. You look just as good as the other doctors said you would. You don't look like you've had cancer."

Ding dong—Is a bell ringing somewhere in the halls of medicine? Maybe—only maybe, of course—there is something to this idea that you are what you eat. I'm convinced that there is. I believe it with every one of those

44 supplement pills I swallow with a tall glass of green tea. It takes a massive assault to deal with this insidious disease. I cannot attack it any other way.

Chapter Sixty-Three

This idea of putting my life in someone else's hands is a tough one for me. I had never seen most of my doctors until I became ill. Now I am supposed to trust them with my money and my life. I don't feel bad or worry about arguing with them or questioning their procedures. I read a story in Guideposts magazine about a woman in a remote village in the mountains. The warrior tribe from the top of the mountain raided her village. They stole her baby. The men of her village formed a party to scale the mountain and rescue her baby. They climbed the mountain and tried to retrieve the baby. The task was too difficult, and they gave up. As they returned to the village, they met the mother of the baby coming down the mountain. She had her baby on her back.

The warriors asked her how did she manage to get her baby. They said they had tried everything they could.

The mother smiled and said, "It's not your baby."

I say to myself, "It is my life, and I will do whatever I need to make it last."

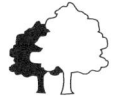

Chapter Sixty-Four

The tumor board decides to wait four more months and do another scan. After our appointment with Dr. Bonebrake, I am okay with that decision. I trust his judgment. He is a bright man who is never threatened by Bill's questions. He says that he welcomes conversations with Bill. His questions make him think again about his recommendations. He is flexible, dedicated and compassionate. This doctor is a gift.

To be honest, however, I never enter his office without a feeling of fear. Inside the room, I sit on the white office bed. Bill sits on a chair and reads a book. My heart pounds as I listen to the sounds outside my door. A shuffle goes by followed by a high noise. I know that shuffle wears a nurse's uniform. Another squeak that halts and then moves on. A tap, tap, tap passes by. I'm sure this time that it is a woman like me. Then the sound I dread and love. It is the solid step of my doctor. I know with the sound of his voice my whole life can change. I have lived this moment an appalling number of times in the last six years. It does not get easier with practice.

Afterword

In October, Bill and I travel to Ghost Ranch in Abiquiu, New Mexico, an incredible stretch of ground that Georgia O'Keeffe immortalized with painting after painting. It is a spiritual place, and there I begin to write.

I find my voice at Ghost Ranch. I hope it will help another woman who belongs to the club that no one wants to join, the ovarian cancer club.

I continue to live and battle this illness. "Through love, all pain will turn to medicine." I read this quote from a poem by Rumi in Anne Lamott's book, *Blue Shoe*. That quote is the story of my battle. Bill, my family, my friends and community taught me this lesson. I hope someone will teach it to you.

There is a Hebrew proverb that says, "From my degradation comes my exultation." That is what cancer gives me—complete and total degradation that is followed by exultation in the sheer joy of being alive—as I write this—seven years, eight months, and twenty-six days after my diagnosis. Death still stands in my face every day, but hope pushes it back. I armor myself with the words of Ralph Waldo Emerson. "What lies behind us and what lies before us are tiny matters compared to what lies within us." If I can leave joy of life, strength of soul, and a piece of God in my love, my legacy to our sons will be complete.

Cancer is like black and white photography. It strips away all that is not essential and illuminates your soul. Cancer takes you right to the heart of what really matters—your family, friends and your fellow man. When I look at other people, I don't just see their clothes, jewelry or hair styles anymore.

With all humility, I think I glimpse their souls. I finally understand what Jesus was trying to do on this earth. He taught us to look at each other's souls and to love as we look. That is the ultimate gift of cancer. When I finish my yoga class, we always say, "Namaste," which means, "I recognize the divine within you."

Never will I ever look at another human being without remembering this gift.

Namaste, my friend.

Gynecological Cancer Resourses

These gynecological cancer resources were particularly helpful to me in my battle. I hope they will help you too.

Nutritional Solutions: www.nutritional solutions@comcast.com
The Health Resource, Inc.: www.thehealthsource.com
Gynecologic Cancer Foundation: www.thegcf.org
Women's Cancer Network: www.wcn.org
Gynecological Cancer Alliance of Springfield, MO: www.gynca.org